Laboratory Manual for

Principles of Animal and Population Genetics

Laboratory Manual for
Principles of Animal and Population Genetics

B. Ramesh Gupta

S. Sai Reddy

COPAL PUBLISHING GROUP

Inspiring for a better future through publishing

Published by Copal Publishing Group
E-143, Lajpat Nagar, Sahibabad,
Distt. Ghaziabad, UP – 201005, India

www.copalpublishing.com

First Published 2017
© Copal Publishing Group, 2017

ISBN: 978-93-83419-51-7 (hard back)
ISBN: 978-93-83419-50-0 (e-book)

Typeset by Bhumi Graphics, New Delhi
Printed and bound by Bhavish Graphics, Chennai

Contents

Preface

The book entitled *Laboratory Manual for Principles of Animal and Population Genetics* is the culmination of the vast experience of offering the courses on Principles of Animal Genetics and Population and Quantitative Genetics to the UG, PG and Ph.D. students of Veterinary Science for more than two decades. The book is written as per the course content of the Unit two of the course on Principles of Animal and Population Genetics under the Department of Animal Genetics and Breeding, as prescribed by the Veterinary Council of India – Minimum Standards of Veterinary Education – Degree Course (B.V.Sc. & A.H.) Regulations, 2015. First five chapters deal with the Principles of Animal Genetics and the next six chapters are devoted to the Population and Quantitative Genetics. For each topic, the class work exercises are explained with simple examples and solving them step by step. Large number of exercises covering various species of animals and plants including humans are provided as Home Work, at the end of each chapter, which may serve as Question Bank.

We immensely thank the students who helped in devising some of the exercises and solving them. We also thank COPAL Publishing Group fortheir keen interest and encouraging us to take up the work and publishing this book. We welcome the suggestions from the readers for further improvement in quality of this book.

B. Ramesh Gupta
S. Sai Reddy

PRACTICAL NO. 1

1.1 CELL DIVISION, CHROMOSOME NUMBER AND KARYOTYPING IN FARM ANIMALS

All living organisms either single-cell like bacteria and yeast or the multicellular plants and animals are made up of cells. Animal cells have a number of structures, each of which has certain functions. The cell membrane surrounds the cell and forms its boundaries. Within the cell lies the protoplasm, mitochondria, ribosomes, Golgi apparatus, centrioles, lysosomes, the nucleus and various other organelles. Inside the cell lie the nucleoli, chromosomes and microtubules and nucleoplasm.

Chromosome definition, structure and function

A chromosome is a thread-like structure of nucleic acids and protein, found in the nucleus of most living cells, carrying the genetic information in the form of genes. The word 'chromosome' was derived from the Greek words *Chroma*, meaning colour, and *soma*, meaning body. The scientist Wilhelm von Waldeyer-Hartz first coined the term *Chromosome* to these structures as they accept dye and take the dark and light patterns when exposed to different stains.

Each chromosome consists of a DNA double helix bearing a linear sequence of genes, coiled and recoiled around aggregated proteins (histones). Their number is fixed among the members of each species but varies from species to species. During cell division, each DNA strand is duplicated and the chromosomes condense to become visible as distinct pairs of chromatids joined at the centromere.

In prokaryotes, the chromosome appears as a circular strand of DNA; and hence, the entire genome is carried on only one chromosome. In viruses, the chromosome appears as a short linear or circular structure consisting of the DNA or RNA molecular often devoid of any proteins. In eukaryotes, the chromosomes appear as thread-like strand, which condense into thicker structures and align on the metaphase plate during Mitosis. Each chromosome occurs in pairs with a characteristic length and banding pattern, since one member of each pair comes from the male parent and the other from the female parent.

Functions of chromosomes

- Chromosomes are essential for cell division and are responsible for replication, division and creation of daughter cells that contain correct sequences of DNA and proteins. Proteins are the most important components of body which are responsible for body muscles and tissues, growth and repair and synthesis of large number of enzymes.

- The normal chromosomes have a single centromere (primary constriction), at which sister chromatids are joined. The centromere is essential for segregation during cell division. During Mitosis, a pair of kinetochores form at each centromere, one attached to each sister chromatid. The microtubules attach to each kinetochore, linking the centromere of a chromosome and two spindle poles. At anaphase, the microtubules pull two sister chromatids toward opposite poles of the spindle. Chromosome fragments that lack a centromere (acentric fragments) do not become attached to the spindle, and so fail to be included in the nuclei of either of the daughter cells.

- The Telomeres of the chromosomes are specialized structures, comprising DNA and protein, which cap the ends of the chromosome and prevent fusing of chromosomes. They ensure complete replication of the extreme ends of chromosomes.

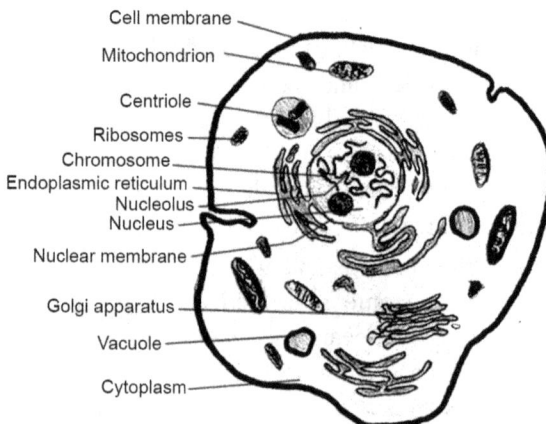

Animal cell diagram
sketch by Abhishkae Sharma

- The normal chromosome number ensures the faithful transmission of genetic information to the offspring generation. Having the wrong number of chromosomes (extra or deficient than normal) has lethal consequences and causes multiple congenital abnormalities because of the imbalance in the levels of gene products encoded on different chromosomes. Having wrong number of sex chromosomes causes multiple congenital abnormalities and sterility.

• The structurally normal chromosomes ensure proper genetic recombination. Chromosomes with structural abnormalities like chromosome breaks, acentric fragments, deletions, duplications, inversions and translocations cause mispaired meiotic recombinations, which lead to abnormal gametogenesis and genetic death of the organisms.

Classification of chromosomes

In unisexual organisms, the chromosomes can be classified into two types: *autosomes* and *allosomes*. Autosomes or somatic chromosomes carry genes which determine the somatic characteristics and have no influence on determining the sex of the organism. On the other hand, the allosomes or sex chromosomes have a significant role in the determination of sex since they carry the genes responsible for sexual characteristics.

In humans and higher mammals, the two allosomes in the female, identical to each other, are designated as XX, while in the male one allosome is identical to that of female and designated as X and the other differing morphologically and genetically is designated as Y. The Y chromosome in most cases is smaller in size than the X chromosome. The Y chromosome in particular determines the male sex and hence it is also designated as *androsome*. Apart from their role in sex determination, the allosomes also have a significant role in sex-linked inheritance.

In birds, moths and butterflies, the allosomes are designated by Z and W chromosomes. The males are homogametic with ZZ and females are heterogametic with ZW chromosome complement.

An organism or cell having only one complete set (n) of chromosomes or genome is called haploid or monoploid while the organism or cell with two sets of chromosomes (2n) or two genomes is known as diploid. The somatic tissues of higher plants and animals are generally diploid in chromosome constitution in contrast with the haploid gametes.

The position of the centromere in the chromosome (which is constant to a given chromosome) varies, i.e. it may occupy different positions. Based on this, four morphological forms have been identified in chromosomes. These are:

(a) **Metacentric:** The centromere occupies a middle position with reference to the length of the chromosome. The two arms are thus almost equal in length. During anaphase movement in cell division, metacentric chromosomes appear 'V' shaped.

(b) **Sub-metacentric:** When the centromere is located at some distance away from the middle region of the chromosome, the position is said to be sub-median, and one arm of the chromosome will be shorter than the other. During anaphase movement, a sub-metacentric chromosome appears 'L' shaped.

(c) **Acrocentric:** In this case, the centromere is positioned almost near one end of the chromosome, i.e. sub-terminal. As a result, one arm of the chromosome will be extremely short and the other very long.

(d) **Telocentric:** When the centromere is situated exactly at one end, the chromosome will be having only one long arm. Telocentric chromosomes are very rare. The truly telocentric chromosomes have been identified in some plants, protozoa and certain mammals.

Type	Position of centromere	Shape	Details
Metacentric	Centre (median)	V-shaped	Equal arms
Sub-metacentric	Near centre (sub-median)	J or L shaped	Two unequal arms
Acrocentric	Near at one end (sub-terminal)	One arm very short and another long	–
Telocentric	Terminal	Rod like	–

Importance of knowing chromosome number in farm animals

Since the number of chromosomes is specific for a species, knowing the number of chromosomes in various species will help characterize, identify and differentiate one from the other.

If the number and the morphology of autosomes and allosomes in normal individuals are known, abnormal individuals carrying the numerical as well as structural chromosome anomalies can be identified and eliminated from the breeding flocks, by which the cytogenetically clean flocks or herds can be maintained. The numerical chromosome anomalies include the ploidy, and structural anomalies consist of deletion, duplication, inversion and translocation.

Mitosis and Meiosis

The cell theory states that each living organism is made up of one or more cells and the new cells arise from pre-existing cells through cell division. The process of formation of new cells from the existing ones can occur through Mitosis and Meiosis, depending on the cell type and the purpose of division.

Mitosis

The Mitosis, which is an equational division, involves the duplication of genetic material and an equal distribution of cell contents into two daughter cells. The cell cycle starts with the interphase, which comprises of growth and DNA duplication, and is followed by a mitotic phase. The mitotic phase then enters into prophase, metaphase, anaphase and telophase. During these phases, the original nucleus dissolves, chromosomes replicate into chromatids, align at the center of the cell and segregate into two new daughter nuclei in the final phase – cytokinesis.

Meiosis

It is a type of cell division which results in the formation of four haploid daughter cells from a single diploid parent cell. During Meiosis, the genetic material is replicated only once, while the nucleus divides twice. The chromosome reduction is achieved through two successive divisions: Meiosis I and Meiosis II. The cell cycle progresses through the stages: interphase I, Meiosis I, cytokinesis, Meiosis II and another event of cytokinesis.

During interphase I, the cell grows and chromosome replicates. In Meiosis I, the pairing of homologous chromosomes takes place and they segregate. Through the cytokinesis, two haploid daughter cells are resulted with intact sister chromatids. The sister chromatids separate during Meiosis II, which is a division similar to Mitosis. The resultant daughter cells are haploid and contain a single set of chromosomes.

The Mitosis and Meiosis can be distinguished with the help of following features:

Mitosis	Meiosis
One parent cell undergoes a single division and gives rise to two daughter cells.	One mother cell undergoes two successive divisions and gives rise to four daughter cells.
A haploid or diploid mother cell can undergo Mitosis.	Only a diploid mother cell can undergo Meiosis.
Daughter cell remains the same as that of its mother cell.	Diploid parent cell is transformed into haploid daughter cells with half the number of chromosomes of its parent cell.
Synapsis and crossing over do not occur.	Synapsis and crossing over between homologous chromosomes occur during Meiosis I.
Genetic identity is retained after mitotic division.	Genetic variation is introduced during meiotic division.
Centromere is split during anaphase, resulting in separation of sister chromatids.	Centromeres and sister chromatid pairs remain intact during Meiosis I but separate during Meiosis II.
Major purpose is vegetative growth and a sexual reproduction.	Major purpose is to facilitate sexual reproduction through gametogenesis.
It occurs in all types of cells.	It occurs only in germinal cells which are involved in sexual reproduction.

X-Y pairing and the pseudoautosomal regions

During Meiosis in females, each chromosome including the X has a fully homologous partner and the two X chromosomes synapse and cross over just like any other pair of homologs. However, in male Meiosis, since the X and Y chromosomes are different from one another, they do not pair in prophase-I. Hence, at anaphase-I, each daughter cell receives one sex chromosome, either X or Y. The X and Y chromosomes pair at the end, rather than along the whole length, due to partial homology between them at the tips of their short arms. The genes in pairing region between X and Y do not show the normal X-linked or Y-linked patterns of inheritance, but segregate like autosomal genes. Because of this behaviour, this region is known as the pseudoautosomal region.

Table 1: Chromosome number (somatic) in some animals and plants

Common name	Genus species	2n Number
Domestic Animals		
African buffalo	*Syncerus caffer caffer*	52
Asiatic Swamp buffalo	*Bubalis bubalis*	50

Common name	Genus species	2n Number
Camel	*Camelus dromedaries*	70
Cat	*Felis catus*	38
Cat	*Felis domesticus*	36
Cattle	*Bos taurus, Bos indicus*	60
Congo buffalo	*Syncerus caffer nanus*	48
Dog	*Canis familiaris*	78
Donkey	*Equus asimus*	62
Goat	*Capra hircus*	60
Horse	*Equus caballus*	64
Pig	*Sus scrofa domesticus*	38
Sheep	*Ovis aries*	54
Birds		
Chicken	*Gallus domesticus*	78
Duck	*Anas platyrhyncha*	80
Pigeon	*Columbia livia*	80
Turkey	*Meleagris gallopavo*	82
Wild Animals		
Alligator	*Alligator missisipiensis*	32
American bison	*Bison bison*	60
Antelope	*Antelocapra Americana*	58
Ass	*Equus asinus*	62
Baboon	*Papio sp.*	42
Cheetah	*Acinonyx jubatus*	38
Chimpanzee	*Pan troglodytes*	24
Common toad	*Bufonidae*	22
Elephant	*Elephas maximus* and *Loxodonta Africana*	56
Fox	*Vulpes vulpes crucigera*	36
Giraffe	*Giraffa camelopardalis*	62
Gorilla	*Gorilla gorilla gorilla*	48
Kangaroo	*Macropus giganteus*	16
Lion	*Panthera leo*	38
Mink	*Mustela vison*	30
Mongoose	*Cynictis penicillata*	36
Musk ox	*Oribus muschatus*	48
Reindeer	*Rangifer tarandus*	70

Common name	Genus species	2n Number
Scorpion	*Pandinus imperator*	4
Snail	*Helix aspersa*	24
Tiger	*Panthera tigris*	38
Wolf	*Canis lupus*	78
Laboratory Animals		
Earth worm	*Lumbricus terrestris*	36
Frog	*Rana pipiens*	26
Guinea pig	*Cavia cobaya*	64
Hamster	*Cricetus cricetus*	20
Hare	*Lepus Linnaeus*	48
Monkey, Rhesus	*Macaca mulata*	48 or 42
Mouse	*Mus musculus*	40
Rabbit	*Oryctolagus cuniculus*	44
Rat	*Rattus norvegicus*	42
Toad	*Xenopus laevis*	34
Flies		
Fruit fly	*Drosophila melanogaster*	8
Grass hopper	*Melanophus differentialis*	24
Honey bee	*Apis mellifera*	32
House fly	*Musca domestica*	12
Mosquito	*Aedes aegypti/ Culex pipiens*	6
Common Plants		
Alfalfa	*Medicago sativa*	32
Apple	*Malus sylvestris*	34, 51
Banana	*Musa paradisiacal*	22 to 88
Barley	*Hordeum vulgare*	14
Bread mold	*Neurospora crassa*	14
Bread wheat	*Triticum aestivum*	42
Cabbage	*Brassica oleracea*	18
Carrot	*Daucus carota*	18
Coffee	*Coffee Arabica*	22 to 88
Cow pea	*Vigna unguiculata*	22
Crucifer	*Arabidopsis thaliana*	10
Cucumber	*Cucumis sativus*	14

Common name	Genus species	2n Number
Maize (Corn)	Zea mays	20
Mango	Mangifera indica	40
Mustard cress	Arabidopsis thaliana	10
Pea (Garden pea)	Pisum sativum	14
Rice	Coryza sativa	24
Radish	Raphanus sativus	18
Snapdragon	Antirrhinum majus	16
Tobacco	Nicotina tabacum	48
Tomato (Husk tomato)	Physalis pubescens	24
Wheat	Triticum gestivum	42
Unicellular green algae	Chlamydomonas reinhardii	34
Yeast, Baker's yeast	Saccharomyces cerevisiae	32
Others		
Fish	Esox lucius	50
Human being	Homo sapiens	46
Lizard	Lacerta vivipara	36
Mule, hinny (hybrids of horse and ass)		63
Silk worm	Bombyx mori	56

The basic number of chromosomes varies with species, and the chromosome number is unrelated to the size of an organism. Most of the species contain the chromosome number ranging from 10 to 40 in their genomes.

Smallest number: The female of a subspecies of the ant, *Myrmecia pilosula*, has one pair of chromosomes per cell. Its male has only one chromosome in each cell. These ants reproduce by a process called haplodiploidy, in which fertilized eggs (diploid) become females, while unfertilized eggs (haploid) develop into males. Hence, the males of this group of ants have, in each of their cells, a single chromosome. The muntjac, a tiny Asian deer, has only three chromosomes in its genome while some species of ferns have many hundreds.

Largest number: In the fern family of plants, the species *Ophioglossum reticulatum* has about 630 pairs of chromosomes, or 1260 chromosomes per cell. The fact that these cells can accurately segregate these enormous numbers of chromosomes during Mitosis is remarkable.

Table 2: Chromosome morphology of common domestic animals

Species	2n	Autosomes				Allosomes	
		Meta centric	Sub-meta centric	Acro centric	Telo centric	X	Y
Cattle							
(a) *Bos indicus*	60	–	–	58	–	Sub-meta	Sub-meta
(b) *Bos taurus*	60	–	–	58	–	Sub-meta	Meta
Buffaloes							
(a) River type	50	–	10	38	–	Large acro	Small acro
(b) Swamp type	48	2	8	36	–	Large acro	Small acro
Sheep	54	6	–	46	–	Longest acro	Acro
Goats	60	–	–	58	–	Acro	Meta/ sub-meta
Pigs	38	–	24	12	–	Sub-meta	Sub-meta
Horse	64	26	–	36	–	Sub-meta	Acro
Rabbit	44	–	34	8	–	Sub-meta	Acro

Karyotyping

The pictoral representation of the chromosomes according to their length and morphology is called karyotype. The process of preparation of karyotype is called karyotyping. The chromosomes are separated from the cells, stained and arranged in order from largest to smallest so that their number and structure can be studied under a microscope. By using a karyotype, characterization of chromosome complement of an individual or a species can be undertaken using the number, form and size of chromosomes.

Major steps in karyotyping

Metaphase cells are required to prepare a standard karyotype and virtually any population of dividing cells could be used. Blood is easily the most frequently sampled tissue, but at times, karyotypes are prepared from cultured skin fibroblasts or bone marrow cells. None of the leukocytes in blood normally divide, but lymphocytes can readily be induced to proliferate, providing a very accessible source of metaphase cells. There are many protocols for preparing a karyotype from peripheral blood lymphocytes, but a rather standard series of steps is involved:

- A sample of blood is drawn and coagulation prevented by addition of heparin.
- Mononuclear cells are purified from the blood by centrifugation through a dense medium that allows red cells and granulocytes to pellet, but retards the mononuclear cells (lymphocytes and monocytes).
- The mononuclear cells are cultured for 3–4 days in the presence of a mitogen like phytohemagglutinin, which stimulates the lymphocytes to proliferate madly.
- At the end of the culture period of 72 hours, when there is a large population of dividing cells, the culture is treated with a drug such as *colcemid*, which disrupts mitotic spindles and prevents completion of Mitosis. This greatly enriches the population of metaphase cells.
- The lymphocytes are harvested and treated briefly with a hypotonic solution (0.075 M potassium chloride). This makes the nuclei swell osmotically and greatly aids in getting preparations in which the chromosomes don't lie on top of one another.
- The swollen cells are fixed, dropped onto a microscope slide and dried.
- Slides are stained after treatment to induce a banding pattern as described above.

Once stained slides are prepared, they are scanned to identify "good" chromosome spreads (i.e. the chromosomes are not too long or too compact and are not overlapping), which are photographed. The photos then are given to kindergarten children, who cut out the images of each chromosome and paste them to a backing sheet in an orderly manner. Alternatively, a digital image of the chromosome can be cut and pasted using a computer. If standard staining was used, the orderly arrangement is limited to grouping like-sized chromosomes together in pairs, whereas if the chromosomes were banded, they can be unambiguously paired and numbered.

The image below shows chromosomes as they are seen on the slide (left panel) and after arrangement (right panel).

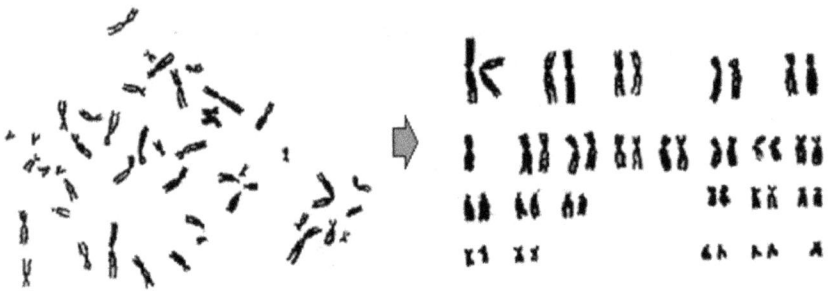

Karyotypes are presented in a standard form. First, the total number of chromosomes is given, followed by a comma and the sex chromosome constitution. This shorthand description is followed by coding of any autosomal abnormalities. A few (simple) examples of this format are:

- A normal male cat: 38, XY
- Horse with three X chromosomes (trisomy X): 65, XXX
- Female dog with increased length of the short (p) arm of chromosome 2: 78, XX, 2p+
- Male pig with a deletion from the long arm (q) of chromosome 10: 38, XY, 10q−

Generally, several metaphases are processed because it's not uncommon for a single spread to artifactually have extra chromosomes or be missing chromosomes. This is particularly important if one is to diagnose an abnormality in an individual. It also allows one to diagnose cases of mosaicism, in which an individual has multiple, cytogenetically distinct populations of cells.

If abnormalities are found in peripheral blood, it is sometimes desirable to determine whether that abnormality is present throughout the individual, and further studies with tissues other than blood can be performed. Also, analysis of diseased tissues can often provide useful information. A prime example of this is the cytogenetic evaluation of cancers, which is not only used diagnostically, but has provided valuable understanding of the pathogenesis of certain types of neoplasia.

HOME WORK

1.1.1   The dog (*Canis familiaris*) has 39 pairs of chromosomes in its somatic cells. (a) How many chromosomes are present in a dog's mature sperm cells? (b) How many sister chromatids are present in a cell that is entering the first meiotic division? (c) In a cell that is entering the second meiotic division?

Solution: (a) If a dog has 39 pairs of chromosomes in its diploid somatic cells, i.e. $2 \times 39 = 78$ chromosomes altogether, a haploid sperm cell, which is an end product of Meiosis, should have half as many chromosomes, i.e. $78/2 = 39$ or one chromosome from each homologous pair. (b) A cell that is entering the first meiotic division has just duplicated its 78 chromosomes. Since each chromosome now has two sister chromatids, altogether $78 \times 2 = 146$ sister chromatids are present in each. (c) A cell which is entering in to second meiotic division has one homologue from each of the $39 \times 2 = 78$ chromatids.

1.1.2   There are 60 chromosomes in somatic cells of the dairy cattle.

(a) How many chromosomes does a cow receive from her father?

(b) How many autosomes are present in a gamete?

(c) How many sex chromosomes are present in ovum?

(d) How many autosomes are present in somatic cells of a bull?

1.1.3   An organism has two homologous pairs of chromosomes: one pair metacentric and the other pair telocentric.

(a) Draw the metaphase plate of the first meiotic division.

(b) Draw the metaphase plate of a second meiotic division.

1.1.4   A plant has eight chromosomes in its root cells: a long metacentric pair, a short metacentric pair, a long telocentric pair and a short telocentric pair. If this plant fertilizes itself, what proportion of the offspring would be expected to have (a) four pair of telocentric chromosomes, (b) one telocentric pair and three metacentric pairs of chromosomes, (c) two metacentric and two telocentric pairs of chromosomes? (d) The garden peas have 14 chromosomes in their somatic cells. How many groups of linked genes occur in this plant?

1.1.5   If a parent having two pairs of chromosomes (I, I, II, II) mates with a parent whose somatic chromosomes are represented by (1,

1, 2, 2), the expected F_1 offspring will have a somatic outfit of chromosomes represented by I, 1, II, 2. (a) What are the different possible combinations when two F_1 individuals mate? (b) If traits borne in the chromosomes represented by the Roman numerals are dominant, how many different appearing organisms may result from this cross? (c) What would be the result if the species possessed eight, instead of four somatic chromosomes?

1.1.6   The following Table shows the number of chromosomes appearing during the first meiotic metaphase, of four different species plants and their F_1 hybrids.

Species or F₁ hybrid	Number of chromosomes	Number of bivalents	Number of univalents
A	20	10	0
B	20	10	0
C	10	5	0
D	10	5	0
A × B	20	0	20
A × C	15	5	5
A × D	15	5	5
C × D	10	0	10

(a) Deduce the chromosomal origin of species A.

(b) How many bivalents and univalents would you expect to observe at meiotic metaphase I in a hybrid between species B and C?

(c) How many bivalents and univalents would you expect to observe at meiotic metaphase I in a hybrid between species D and B?

1.1.7   The *Drosophila virilis* fly has a diploid chromosome number of 12 (6 pairs altogether). How many chromatids and chromosomes are present in the following stages of cell   division?

(a) Metaphase of Mitosis, (b) Metaphase I of Meiosis, (c) Metaphase II of Meiosis

1.1.8   The human sperm cell contains 23 chromosomes. (a) How many chromosomes would be present in a spermatogonial cell about to enter Meiosis? (b) How many chromatids would be present in a spermatogonial cell at metaphase I of Meiosis? (c) How many would be present at metaphase II?

1.1.9   Two highly inbred strains of guinea pigs, one with black fur (G) and the other with gray (g) fur were crossed and all the offspring obtained were of black fur. Predict the outcome of intercrossing the offspring.

1.1.10   A G1-stage human chromosome contains a single DNA molecule. How many DNA molecules would be present in the chromosomes of the nucleus of (a) an egg, (b) a sperm, (c) diploid somatic cell in G1 stage, (d) diploid somatic cell in G2 stage and (e) a primary oocytes?

Ans: A human haploid cell contains 23 chromosomes and a diploid cell contains 46 chromosomes or 23 pairs of homologues. If replication chromosomes contain a single DNA molecule, post-replication chromosomes will contain two DNA molecules, one in each of two chromatics. Thus normal human eggs and sperm contains 23 chromosomes; diploid somatic cells contain 46 and 92 chromosomal DNA molecules at stages G1 and G2 respectively, and a primary oocytes contains 92 such DNA molecules.

1.1.11   The RNA extracted from TMV was found containing 35 percent cytosine, i.e. 35% of the bases were cytosine. Is it possible to predict what percentage of the total bases is adenine? (Ans: No, TMV RNA is single stranded).

1.1.12   In a DNA sample isolated from the cells of staphylococcus aurius, it was found that 45% of the bases are cytosine. Predict the percentage of adenine bases.

1.1.13   If a strand of DNA of a bacterial DNA has the sequence 5'-TGACGTGT-3', what is the base sequence of the complementary strand?

1.2 MONOHYBRID INHERITANCE

The Mendel's Laws of Inheritance can be defined as follows.

1. **Law of Segregation**

    The allelic genes in a zygote do not blend or contaminate each other, but segregate and pass into different gametes.

2. **Law of Independent and Random Assortment**

    The genes in any one pair of allele segregate independently of those in other pairs of alleles.

    The F_2 phenotypic ratio = 3:1

    The F_2 genotypic ratio = 1:2:1

    Monohybrid test cross ratio = 1:1

CLASS WORK

1. In garden pea, tall plant is dominant over dwarf plant.

    (a) If a homozygous tall is crossed with a dwarf plant, describe (i) the genotypes and phenotypes of F_1 and F_2 progeny and (ii) the genotypes and phenotypes of the test cross progeny.

    (b) A tall plant is crossed with a dwarf plant. In the progeny, about one half of the progeny are tall and the remaining one-half are dwarf. Determine the genotypes of the tall and dwarf plants.

    Answer:

    a. (i) Parents: Phenotype: Tall × Dwarf

    Genotype: TT × tt

    Gametes formed: T   T   t   t

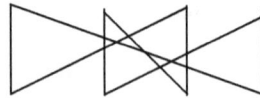

    F_1 offspring: Tt   Tt   Tt   Tt

    All tall plants

    F_2 Tall   ×   Tall

                     Tt   ×   Tt

Gametes formed: T   t   T   t

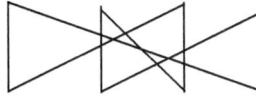

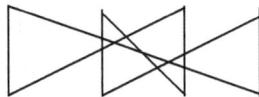

F$_2$ offspring: TT   Tt   Tt   tt
                      Tall Tall Tall Dwarf
F$_2$ phenotypic ratio: 3 tall : 1 dwarf
F$_2$ genotypic ratio: 1 TT   :   2 Tt   :   1 tt
                 Homozygous Heterozygous Homozygous
                      tall   tall   dwarf

a. (ii) Test cross: Test cross is crossing of the F$_1$ with homozygous recessive individual.

Parents: Phenotype: Tall   × Dwarf
             Genotype: Tt   ×   tt
             Gametes formed: T   t   t   t

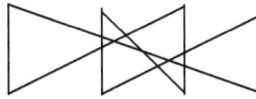

Offspring: Tt   Tt   tt   tt
Phenotypes: Tall   Tall   dwarf   dwarf
Test cross ratio Tall : dwarf = 1 : 1
b. Parents: Phenotype: Tall   × Dwarf
              Genotype: TT or Tt ×   tt
Case (a): Let the parent's genotype be TT. Then,
Gametes formed: T   T   t   t

Offspring: Tt   Tt   Tt   Tt
Phenotypes: Tall   Tall   Tall   Tall
                        all plants tall
Therefore, the genotype of the tall parent cannot be TT

Case (b): Let the parent's genotype be Tt. Then,

Gametes formed: T   t   t   t

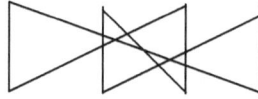

Offspring:	Tt	tt	tt	Tt
Phenotypes:	Tall	dwarf	dwarf	Tall

Phenotypic ratio: 1 tall : 1 dwarf

Therefore, the genotypes of the tall and dwarf parents are Tt and tt, respectively.

2. In cattle, the polled or hornless condition, P is dominant over the horned, p. A polled bull is bred to three cows. With cow A, which is horned, a polled calf is produced; with cow B, also horned, a horned calf is produced; with cow C, which is polled, a horned calf is produced. Find out the genotypes of the four parents and what further offspring, in what proportions, would you expect from these matings?

    The possible genotype of the polled bull in question can be either PP or Pp since the P allele is completely dominant over the p and heterozygous polled, phenotypically, cannot be distinguished from the homozygous polled.

Polled bull (PP or Pp) × Cow-A (horned, pp) → Polled calf (Pp only since p allele has come from the horned cow, and P necessarily from the bull)

Polled bull (PP or Pp) × Cow-B (horned, pp) → Horned calf (pp, one 'p' allele has come from the horned cow, while the other recessive allele 'p' has come from the bull in question. Since the calf is horned (pp), the bull must be a heterozygous (carrier) polled. Therefore, genotype of polled bull must be 'Pp' but not 'PP').

Polled bull (PP or Pp) × Cow-C (polled, PP or Pp) → Horned calf (pp, one 'p' allele come from the horned cow and the other 'p', necessarily from the bull, to make the calf, a horned one)

    If the genotype of polled bull is PP, then the birth of a horned calf is not possible with cow B, which is horned. Therefore, the genotype of bull is Pp and those of the cows A, B and C are pp, pp and Pp, respectively.

HOME WORK

1.2.1   In pea plants, the green pods are dominant to yellow pods. If a number of crosses are made between green pod (GG) and yellow pod (gg) plants, what will be the phenotypes and genotypes of the F_1 and F_2 plants?

1.2.2   In garden peas, the tall pea plants (T) are dominant over the dwarf (t).

   (a) If a pure tall plant is crossed with a pure dwarf one, what will be the appearance of the offspring?

   (b) What results are expected:
       (i) When these hybrids are crossed?
       (ii) When the hybrid tall plants are crossed back to the dwarf parent?
       (iii) When the tall hybrids are crossed back to the pure tall parents?

   (c) What kind of gametes will be produced by:
       (i) Pure tall parents, (ii) hybrid tall parents and (iii) dwarf parents?

   (d) A dwarf parent is crossed with a tall parent, producing about half tall and half white. What are the genotypes of the parents?

   (e) What will be the appearance of the crosses: TT × tt; Tt × tt; TT × Tt; Tt × Tt?

   (f) If two tall parents produce about three-fourths tall offspring, what is their genotype?

   (g) How to determine whether the tall plants are pure or hybrid?

   (h) How to determine whether the dwarf plants are pure or hybrid?

1.2.3   The red fruit colour in tomatoes is dominant to yellow one. If a homozygous red-fruited tomato plant is crossed with the yellow-fruited one, determine the appearance of the following.

   (a) F_1 offspring
   (b F_2 offspring
   (c) Offspring of the cross of F_1 back to the red parent
   (d) Offspring of the cross of F_1 back to the yellow parent

1.2.4   In man, brown eyes (B) are dominant over blue eyes (b).

(a) What phenotypes of the offspring with respect to their eye colour are expected from the following crosses?

(i) BB × bb, (ii) Bb × Bb, (iii) Bb × bb, (iv) Bb × BB

(b) A brown-eyed (B) man marries a blue-eyed (b) woman and all the children born to them were brown eyed. What are the genotypes of the parents and offspring?

(c) A blue-eyed man (b) whose parents were brown eyed (B) marries a brown-eyed woman. They have produced one blue-eyed child. Find out the genotypes of all the individuals?

1.2.5   A cow has two calvings. Find out the probability that it has (a) one male and one female calf, (b) both males and (c) both females (expand the binomial equation $(p + q)^2$).

1.2.6   A cross was made between homozygous tall (TT) and dwarf (tt) pea plants. What will be the appearance of F_1 and F_2, of the offspring of a cross of F_1 with tall and dwarf parents?

1.2.7   In cats, the long hair is recessive (l) to short hair (L). (a) A true breeding (homozygous) short-haired male is mated to a long-haired female. What will their kittens look like? (b) Two cats were mated. One of the parent cats is long haired. The litter which results contains two short-haired and three long-haired kittens. What does the second parent look like and what is its genotype?

1.2.8   A family consists of a father, mother and their six children. Three of the children have the attached earlobes (recessive) like their father and the other three have free earlobes like their mother. What are the genotypes of the father, mother and their offspring?

1.2.9   In guinea pigs, the gene B causes the coat colour to be black and b, white. A carrier black male is mated to white female.

(a) If the mating produces two offspring, what is the probability that one will be black and one white.

(b) If it has produced six offspring, what is the probability that three are blacks and three whites? (Apply expansion of binomial equation $(a + b)^2$ and $(a + b)^6 = p^6 + 6\,p^5q + 15p^4q^2 + 20p^3q^3 + 15p^2q^4 + 6pq^5 + q^6$)

1.2.10   In humans, about 80% of the population can taste the chemical phenolthiocarbamide (PTC) and other 20% cannot. This characteristic is governed by a single gene with two alleles: a tasting allele and a non-testing allele. Which allele is dominant?

1.2.11   In guinea pigs, rough coat (R) is dominant over smooth coat (r). A rough-coated guinea pig is bred to a smooth one, giving eight rough and seven smooth progeny in the F_1. (a) What are the genotypes of the parents and their offspring? (b) If one of the F_1 animals is mated to its rough parent, what progeny would you expect?

1.2.12   Albinism, the total lack of pigment, is due to a recessive gene. A man and a woman plan to marry and wish to know the probability of their having any albino children. What could you tell them if (a) both are normally pigmented, but each has one albino parent; (b) the man is an albino, the woman is normal, but her father is an albino; (c) the man is an albino and the woman's family includes no albinos for at least three generations.

1.2.13   Some people are able to taste the chemical phenylthiocarbamide (PTC), whereas others cannot. From the marriages of two tasters, the children are both tasters and non-tasters. From the marriage of two nontasters, all the children are nontasters. What type of inheritance is involved?

1.2.14   A woman has a rare abnormality of the eyelids called *ptosis*, which makes it impossible for her to open her eyes completely. The condition has been found to depend on a single dominant gene (P). The woman's father had *ptosis*, but her mother had normal eyelids. Her father's mother had normal eyelids. (a) What are the probable genotypes of the woman, her father and mother? (b) What proportion of her children will be expected to have *ptosis* if she marries a man with normal eyelids?

1.2.15   In Drosophila, a female with sepia eyes was crossed to a male with red eyes. All the F_1 had red eyes. In the F_2, there were 224 red-eyed flies and 72 sepia-eyed flies.

(a) How does sepia eye appear to be inherited?
(b) What are the genotypes of the parents?
(c) What gametes are produced by the parents?
(d) What is the genotype of the F_1?
(e) What gametes do the F_1 produce?
(f) What is the genotypic ratio in the F_2?

1.2.16   In cattle, the polled (P) condition is dominant to horned (p) phenotype. A polled Ongole bull was crossed to 3 Ongole cows.

(a) With cow-A, which is horned, a horned calf is produced.

(b) With cow-B, which is polled, a horned calf is produced.

(c) With cow-C, which is horned, a polled calf is produced.

Determine the genotypes of the bull and cows A, B and C and what phenotypic ratios do you expect in the offspring of these three matings.

1.2.17 Deafness in dogs is an inherited disorder controlled by a single locus with two alleles. A kennel breeder has done matings between three normal dogs namely A, B and C. Mating of female N with male C produced 15 puppies; all were normal. Mating of female B with male C produced 4 normal and 1 deaf puppy.

(a) Find out whether the allele for deafness is dominant or recessive?

(b) If the breeder wished to eliminate the allele for deafness from his kennel and had the opportunity to sell female A, female B and male C for house pets, which animals should he sell?

1.2.18 In man, brown eyes (B) are dominant over blue eyes (b).

(a) What phenotypes are expected with respect to the eye colour in the following crosses:

(i) BB × bb, (ii) Bb × Bb, (iii) Bb × bb, (iv) Bb × BB

(b) A brown-eyed man marries a blue-eyed woman and they have all brown-eyed children. Find out the genotypes of the parents and children?

(c) A blue-eyed man, whose parents were brown eyed, marries a brown-eyed woman. They have one blue-eyed child. Find out the genotypes of all the individuals involved.

(d) Two brown-eyed individuals, each of whom had a blue-eyed parent marry, what is the probability that the first child will have brown eyes? If the brown-eyed child results, what is the probability that the child will be heterozygous? What is the probability that this couple will have three children with blue eyes?

1.2.19 In a sib'ship of three children work out the probabilities for the different combination of boys and girls. (Ans: probability of all being boys = ½; probability of all being girls = ½; probability of two boys and one girls = 3/8 and probability of two girls and one boy = 3/8).

1.2.20 Four children are born on a particular day in a certain hospital. What is the probability that: (a) all four are girls (b) all four are of the same sex, i.e. either all males or all females and (c) three boys and one girl?

(Ans: (a) 1/16, (b) 1/8, (c) ¼)

1.2.21 If eight babies are born on a given day: (a) What is the chance that four will be boys and four girls? (b) What is the chance that all eight will be girls? (c) What combination of boys and girls among the eight babies is most likely? What is the chance that at least one baby will be a girl? (d) In a family of five children, what is the chance that at least two are girls?

1.2.22 In humans, albinism is inherited as an autosomal recessive trait. A normally pigmented woman marries an albino man and they have 7 children, all normally pigmented. What are the genotypes of the parents and of the children?

1.2.23 A normally pigmented man whose father was an albino marries an albino woman whose parents were both normally pigmented. They have three children, two normally pigmented and one albino. Find out the genotypes of the parents and children.

1.2.24 Phenylketonuria is a metabolic disease in humans caused by a recessive allele, k. If two heterozygous carriers for the allele marry and plan a family of five children, (a) what is the probability that all their children will be unaffected? (b) What is the chance that four children will be unaffected and one affected with phenylketonuria? (c) What is the chance that at least three children will be unaffected? (d) What is the chance that the first child will be an unaffected girl?

(Answers: (a) Use multiplicative rule of probability. When two heterozygotes are crossed, probability of unaffected (p) is ¾ and affected (q) is ¼ and the probability of a child being boy or girl is ½. For one child probability of unaffected (p) is ¾ and for all five to be affected, the probability is $(3/4)^5 + (1/4)^0 = 0.237$. (b) The probability of four children unaffected and one affected can be worked out by expanding the binomial equation $[5!/(4! 1!) \times (3/4)^4 \times (1/4)^1] = 0.399$. (c) To find probability that at least three children will be unaffected is the sum of probabilities of 5 unaffected 0 affected + 4 unaffected 1 affected + 3 unaffected 2 affected $= 0.237 + 0.399 + 0.264 = 0.900$. (d) To work out the probability of first children being an unaffected girl, use the multiplication theorem P (unaffected girl child) = (probability of unaffected child) × (probability of girl child) = (3/4) × (½) = 3/8.

1.2.25   The wild mice typically have a gray-brown or agouti fur colour. But one of the laboratory strains had yellow fur. In a breeding experiment, one yellow male was mated to several agouti females and the matings produced a total of 40 progeny out of which 22 were agouti and 18 yellow. The agouti F_1 females were intercrossed with each other to produce F_2 generation, all of which were agouti. Similarly, the F_1 yellow mice were intercrossed with each other but their F_2 progeny segregated into two classes of which 30 were agouti and 54 yellow. Subsequent crosses between yellow F_2 animals also segregated yellow and agouti progeny. Explain the genetic basis of these coat colour differences in that flock.

1.2.26   In a lab animal breeding experiment, a geneticist crossed wild gray coloured mice with white (albino) mice. All the progeny (F_1) obtained were gray, which were then intercrossed to produce an F_2, which consisted of 396 gray and 144 mice. Explain these results, diagram the crosses and compare the results with the predictions of the hypothesis.

1.2.27   Conduct a chi-square test to determine whether an observed ratio of 40 tall : 10 dwarf pea plants is consistent with an expected ratio of 1:1 from the cross Dd × dd.

1.3 DIHYBRID INHERITANCE

The Mendel's Law of independent assortment (2nd law) states that the allele pairs separate independently during the formation of gametes. This means that traits are transmitted to offspring independently of one another.

Mendel formulated this principle after performing dihybrid crosses between the plants that differed in two traits, such as seed color and pod color. After these plants were allowed to self-pollinate, he noticed that the same ratio 9:3:3:1 appeared among the offspring. Mendel concluded that traits are transmitted to offspring independently. A cross between two parents which differ by two pairs of alleles (AABB × aabb) is known as a '*dihybrid cross*' and an individual heterozygous for two pairs of alleles (AaBb) is known as a '*dihybrid*'.

The dihybrid inheritance can be explained by an example in which the plants with yellow seed colour, round seed shape were crossed with the one producing green seed colour and wrinkled seed shape. The gene for yellow seed (Y) colour and round seed shape (R) were dominant over the green seed colour (y) and wrinkled seed surface (r). In F_1 generation, all plants were yellow and round. In F_2 generation, the phenotypic ratio will be 9:3:3:1.

CLASS WORK

1. In garden pea, yellow seed colour (Y) is dominant over green (y) and round seed shape (R) is dominant over wrinkled (r). The two character pairs segregate independently.

   (a) If a homozygous yellow round plant is crossed with green wrinkled one, what will be the appearance of F_1 and F_2? What will be the appearance of the offspring of a cross of F_1 × yellow round parent and of F_1 × green wrinkled parent?

   (b) Determine the genotypes of parents in each of the following crosses:

      (i) A yellow round × green wrinkled cross gave 62 yellow round and 59 yellow wrinkled.

      (ii) Yellow wrinkled × yellow wrinkled gave 59 yellow wrinkled and 21 green wrinkled offspring.

      (iii) Yellow round × yellow wrinkled gave three-eighths yellow round, three-eighths yellow wrinkled, one-eighths green round and one-eighths green wrinkled offspring.

(a) Parents: Yellow, round × Green, wrinkled

   Genotype: YYRR yyrr

Gametes: YR yr

F_1 genotype: YyRr

F_1 phenotype: All yellow, round

F_1 gametes:YR Yr yR yr × YR Yr yR yr

F_2 offspring:

♀ / ♂	YR	Yr	yR	yr
YR	YYRR	YYRr	YyRR	YyRr
Yr	YYRr	YYrr	YyRr	Yyrr
yR	YyRR	YyRr	yyRR	yyRr
yr	YyRr	Yyrr	yyRr	yyrr

F_2 phenotypic ratio: Yellow round = 9/16

   Yellow wrinkled = 3/16

   Green round = 3/16

   Green wrinkled = 1/16

Cross of F_1 parent × yellow round plant

Parents:

Phenotype: Yellow round × yellow round

Genotype: YyRr × YYRR

Gametes: YR Yr yR yr × YR

Offspring:

♀ / ♂	YR	Yr	yR	yr
YR	YYRR Yellow round	YYRr Yellow round	YyRR Yellow round	YyRr Yellow round

Offspring phenotype: All yellow round

Cross of F$_1$ parent × Green wrinkled plant

Parents:

Phenotype: Yellow round × Green wrinkled

Genotype: YyRr × yyrr

Gametes: YR Yr yR yr × yr

Offspring:

♀ / ♂	YR	Yr	yR	yr
Yr	YyRr Yellow round	Yyrr Yellow wrinkled	yyRr Green round	yyrr Green wrinkled

Offspring phenotype: yellow round: yellow wrinkled: green round: green wrinkled = 1:1:1:1 (It is nothing but the test cross).

(b) (i) Parents: Yellow round   ×   Green wrinkled

(Y_R_)   (yyrr)

Offspring: 62 yellow round

59 yellow wrinkled

Since all the offspring are of the yellow seed colour, the parent in question must be homozygous for yellow gene. As there are wrinkled offspring, the parent must be heterozygous round at this locus.

Therefore, the genotypes of the parents are YyRr and yyrr.

(ii) Parents: Yellow wrinkled   ×   yellow wrinkled

(Y_rr)   (Y_rr)

Offspring: 59 yellow wrinkled (73.8%)

21 green wrinkled (26.2%)

The genes for yellow and green seed colour are segregating nearly at 3:1 ratio. Therefore, the two parents must be heterozygous yellow. The genotypes of the parents are Yyrr and Yyrr.

(iii) Parents: Yellow round   ×   yellow wrinkled

(Y_R_)   (Y_rr)

Offspring: 3/8 yellow round

3/8 yellow wrinkled

1/8 green round

1/8 green wrinkled

Within the yellow colour, the round and wrinkled genes segregated in a ratio of 1:1. Therefore, the yellow round parent must be heterozygous for shape of the seed, i.e. Y_Rr.

Similarly, within the shape of the seed (without round and within wrinkled), the genes for yellow and green are segregating independently at 3:1 ratio. Therefore, both the parents must be heterozygous for this locus.

Hence, the genotypes of the parents are YyRr and Yyrr.

HOME WORK

1.3.1   How many F_1 gametes, F_2 genotypes and F_2 phenotypes would be expected from?

(a) AA × aa

(b) AABB × aabb

(c) AABBCC × aabbcc

(d) What general formula can be applied for F_1 gametes, F_2 genotypes and F_2 phenotypes?

1.3.2   How many phenotypic classes are produced by a test cross in which one parent is heterozygous for (a) two pairs of genes, (b) three pairs of genes, (c) four pairs of genes and (d) n pairs of genes?

1.3.3   When a pea plant of genotype AaBb produces gametes, what proportion will be Ab? (Assume that the two genes are independent). Choose the correct answer from the following possible answers: ¾, ½, 9/16, none or ¼.

1.3.4   What conclusions could you reach about the parents if the offspring had phenotypes in the following proportions?

(a) 3:1 (b) 1:1 (c) 9:3:3:1 (d) 1:1:1:1

1.3.5   In Drosophila, the gene for black body colour (B) is in the second chromosome and that for sepia eye colour (s) is in the third chromosome. A black male (BBSS) is crossed with a sepia female (bbss). (a) What results are expected in F_1 and F_2 generations? (b) What might be expected if these two genes were in the same chromosome?

1.3.6   In sorghum, the blackish purple colour (P) is dominant over the brown (pp). The gene Q has no phenotypic expression of its own but modifies the blackish colour into reddish when in combination with gene P. What will be genotypes and phenotypes and in what proportion of the offspring of the following crosses?

(a) PpQq × PpQq, (b) PPqq × ppQQ, (c) PPQq × Ppqq, (d) Ppqq × ppQq

1.3.7   In pea plants, round seed (R) is dominant over wrinkled (r) and tall (T) over the dwarf (t). Find out the appearance of the offspring of the following in crosses in F_1 and F_2?

(a) RRTT × rrtt, (b) rrTT × RRtt, (c) RRTt × rrtt, (d) Rrtt × rrTt

1.3.8   Find out the probability of occurrence of offspring of following genotypes from the dihybrids cross mating of BbPp × BbPp with an assumption that the two loci assort independently.

(a) BbPp, (b) Bbpp, (c) bbpp

1.3.9   What is the probability of obtaining the following phenotypes among the progeny of dihybrid parents for conditions of horns and coat colour (polled, P; horned, p; Black coat B; and Red coat, b)?

Red polled; Red horned; Black polled and Black horned

(Ans: Apply multiplication law after working out individual probabilities by branching method.)

1.3.10   In garden peas, yellow seed colour (Y) is dominant over green (y), and round seed shape (R) is dominant over wrinkled (r). The two characters segregate independently. Find out the genotypes of the parents in the following crosses.

(a) A green wrinkled offspring is obtained from a cross of yellow round × yellow wrinkled. What other offspring may be expected from this cross and in what proportion?

(b) A yellow round × green wrinkled cross gave 62 yellow round and 59 yellow wrinkled.

(c) Yellow wrinkled × yellow wrinkled gave 59 yellow wrinkled and 21 green wrinkled offspring.

(d) Yellow round × yellow wrinkled gave three-eighths yellow round, three eighths yellow wrinkled, one-eighths green round and one-eighths green wrinkled offspring.

(e) Yellow round × green wrinkled gave one yellow round, 1 yellow wrinkled, 1 green round and 1 green wrinkled offspring.

(f) Yellow round × yellow round gave 63 yellow round, 21 yellow wrinkled, 21 green round and 7 green wrinkled.

1.3.11 Normal hearing depends on the presence of at least one dominant of each of two pairs of genes, D and E. If you examined the collective progeny of a large number of DdEe × DdEe marriages, what phenotypic ratio would you expect to find?

1.3.12 In Jimsonweed, the purple flower (P) is dominant to white (p) and spiny pod (S) is dominant to smooth (s). What progeny would you expect from the following Jimsonweed cross?

(a) PPss × ppSS, (b) PpSS × ppss, (c) PpSs × PpSS, (d) PpSs × PpSs, (e) PpSs × Ppss, (f) PpSs × ppss

1.3.13 In mice, the gene for coloured fur (C) is dominant over its allele (c) for white. The gene for normal behavior (V) is dominant over (v) for waltzing. Give the probable genotypes of the parent mice (each pair was mated repeatedly and produced the following results):

(a) Coloured normal mated with white normal produced 29 coloured normal and 10 coloured waltzers.

(b) Coloured normal mated with coloured normal produced 38 coloured normal, 15 coloured waltzers, 11 white normal and 4 white waltzers.

(c) Coloured normal mated with white waltzer produced 8 coloured normal, 7 coloured waltzers, 9 white normal and 6 white waltzers.

1.3.14 The short-hair (S) and pigmented skin (P) in guinea pigs are dominant over the long hair (s) and albino (p). In a cross of short-haired pigmented guinea pig with long-haired albino one, all the hybrid offspring were alike, i.e. short-haired pigmented. When these hybrids are interbred (SsPp × SsPp), there are four possible combinations of pairs so far as the appearance (phenotype) of the resulting animals is concerned:

Gametes	SP = Shirt-haired, pigmented	Like grandparents
	sp = Long-haired, albino	
	Sp = short-haired, albino	New combinations
	sP = Long-haired, pigmented	

(a) Multiply SP + sp + Sp + sP (possible gametes of one parent) by SP + sp + Sp + sP (possible gametes of other parent). There will be 4 apparent kinds (phenotypes), 9 kinds that are actually different (genotypes) and 16 combinations.

(b) Indicate all the phenotypes and genotypes

1.3.15 In man, assume that brown eyes (B) are dominant over blue eyes (b); and that right-handedness (R) dominates the left-handedness (r).

(a) What offspring may be expected from the marriage of a right-handed, blue-eyed man, whose father was left-handed, with a brown-eyed woman from a family in which all the members have been brown-eyed for several generations?

(b) A brown-eyed, right-handed man marries a right-handed, brown-eyed woman. Their first child is blue-eyed and left-handed. If other children are born to this couple, what probably will be their appearance with respect to these two traits?

(c) A right-handed, blue-eyed man marries a right-handed, brown-eyed woman. They have two children, one left handed and brown eyed and the other right handed and blue eyed. By a later marriage with another woman, who is also right handed and brown eyed, this man has nine children, all of whom are right handed and brown eyed. Then, (i) what is the genotype of this man; (ii) what is the genotype of his first wife? (iii) And of his second wife?

1.3.16 Black coat colour in Cocker Spaniels is governed by a dominant allele B and red coat colour by its recessive allele b; solid pattern is governed by the dominant allele of an independently assorting locus S and spotted pattern by its recessive allele s. A solid black male is mated to a solid red female and produced a litter of six pups: two solid black, two solid red, one black and white and one red and white. Determine the genotypes of the parents.

1.3.17 In Drosophila, vestigial wings and ebony body colour are controlled by two recessive genes, while long wings and grey body colour by dominant genes. What will be genotypes and phenotypes of the F_1 and F_2 offspring from a cross between homozygous vestigial ebony female and homozygous long-winged grey males?

1.3.18 In man, spotted skin (S) is dominant to non-spotted (ss), and wooly hair (W) is dominant to non-wooly (w). Both S and W segregate independently. What will be genotype and phenotype of the children expected from a marriage of man and woman having Ssww and ssWw genotypes?

1.3.19 Tall tomato plants are produced by the action of a dominant allele D and dwarf plants by its recessive allele d. Hairy stems are produced by a dominant gene H and hairless stems by its recessive allele h. A dihybrid tall, hairy plant is test crossed. The F_1 progeny were observed to be 118 tall, hairy: 121 dwarf, hairless: 112 tall, hairless: 109 dwarf, hairy.

(a) Show the crossings in the form of a diagram.

(b) What is the ratio of tall: dwarf and hairy: hairless?

(c) Find out whether these two loci assorting independently of one another?

1.3.20 The ebony (e) body colour in Drosophila is produced by the recessive and wild-type (gray) body colour by its dominant allele (e+). Vestigial wings are governed by a recessive gene (vg) and normal wing size (wild type) by its dominant allele (vg+). If wild-type dihybrid flies are crossed and produced 256 progeny, how many of these progeny flies are expected in each phenotypic class?

1.3.21 Short hair in rabbits is controlled by a dominant gene (L) and long hair by its recessive allele (l). Black hair results from the action of the dominant genotype (B_) and brown from the recessive genotype (bb).

(a) In crosses between dihybrid short, black and homozygous short, brown rabbits, what genotypic and phenotypic ratios are expected among their progeny?

(b) Determine the expected genotypic and phenotypic ratios in progeny from the cross LlBb × LlBb.

1.3.22 In garden peas, the genes C and P are essential for coloured flowers. In the absence of either or both (C-pp, ccP-, ccpp) results in white flowers.

(a) What will be the flower colour of the offspring in the following crosses and in what proportion?

(i) Ccpp × ccPp, (ii) ccpp × CcPp, (iii) CcPp × Ccpp, (iv) CcPp × CcPp

(b) Find the genotypes and phenotypes of the offspring and parents from the following:

(i) A purple flowering plant crossed with a white one produced 20 purple and 21 white.

(ii) A white flowering plant crossed with a purple one produced three-eighth purple and five-eighth white offspring.

(iii) A purple flowering plant crossed with a white one produced 50% purple and 50% white offspring.

(iv) A white flowering plant crossed with another white produced three-fourth white and one-fourth purple offspring.

(v) A purple crossed with another purple produced six-eighth purple and two-eighth white progenies.

1.3.23 In human beings, the ability to taste a compound called *phenylthiourea* is inherited. To about 70% of the people of North America, this compound tastes very bitter; while the remaining 30% find it tasteless, called 'non-tasters', recessive (tt). Assume that this allelic pair is independent of albinism in genetic transmission.

(a) Two tasters, normally pigmented, have an albino son and a nontaster daughter, not albino. What is the chance that the albino son is a taster? That the nontaster daughter is a carrier of albinism?

(b) If a non-taster, non-albino daughter in the above problem marries a taster man, normally pigmented, whose mother was non-taster albino, what chance has their child of being a taster? An albino? A taster-albino?

1.3.24 In dog, dark coat colour (D) is dominant over albino (d) and short hair (S) over long hair (s). Both genes are segregating independently. What phenotypic ratios are expected from following matings?

(a) DdSs × DdSs, (b) DDSs × Ddss, (c) DdSs × ddss, (iv) DdSs × Ddss

1.3.25 Normal cloven-footed condition in swine is caused by a recessive, m, and the mule-footed phenotype by its dominant allele, M. Coat colour is governed by another locus: white by dominant allele, B, and black by its recessive allele, b, A mule-footed, white boar (male pig) is mated to a mule-footed, black sow (female pig) and produced a litter containing: mule-footed, white; mule-footed, black; cloven-footed, white; and cloven-footed, black offspring. What are the genotypes of the parents? (Ans: male is Mm Bb and female is Mm bb.)

1.3.26 In mice, the allele for coloured fur (C) is dominant over the allele for white fur (c). The allele, V for normal behaviour is dominant over the allele, v, for waltzing behaviour (a form of dis-coordination). Both the loci assort independent of each other.

(a) A coloured, normal behaviour female mated with a white, waltzing male always produced coloured, normal progeny. What is the most probable genotype of the female parent?

(b) A coloured, normal behaviour male mated with a white, waltzing female produced coloured, normal and coloured, waltzing offspring. What is the probable genotype of the male parent used in this cross?

(Ans: (a) The female parent is CCVV; (b) the male parent is CCVv.)

1.3.27 In rabbits, the coat pattern is controlled by a single locus with two alleles: 'S' for spotted-coat and 's' for solid-coat. The colour of coat is controlled by an independently assorting locus: B for black coat and b for brown coat. All the progeny produced by mating of a solid black male to a spotted brown female were spotted black.

(a) What is the genotype of the progeny?

(b) What would be the probable phenotypic ratio(s) of the F_2 progeny obtained from inter-se-mating of F_1 (i.e., mating among the spotted black F_1)?

(Ans: (a) SsBb; (b) Spotted black = 9; Solid black = 3; Spotted brown = 3; Solid brown = 1)

1.3.28 A laboratory strain of mice contained *agouti* (gray-brown) and yellow-coloured animals. A single yellow male was mated to several agouti females. The matings produced both agouti and yellow progeny. The F_1 agouti mice were crossed among themselves (inter-se-mated) to produce the F_2 generation, all of which were agouti. The inter-se-mating of yellow F_1 mice produced the progeny (F_2) which showed both agouti and yellow fur. Inter-crossing of yellow F_1 mice produced the progeny (F_2), which showed both agouti and yellow fur. Inter-crossing among F_2 yellow mice produced both yellow and agouti progeny. Assume the trait fur-colour is controlled by a single locus with two alleles.

(a) Which of the alleles is dominant?

(b) What are the probable genotypes of the parents?

(c) What could be the genotypes of the F_1 agouti and yellow mice?

(Ans: (a) Yellow fur due to dominant allele, Y; and agouti due to its recessive allele, y; (b) Yellow male parent is Yy and the agouti female parent is yy; (c) The F_1 agouti and yellow would be yy and Yy.)

1.3.29 Feather colour in pigeons is controlled by a single gene with two alleles. The allele for red colour, B, is dominant to the allele for brown colour, b. A red male pigeon that had one red parent and one brown parent is mated with a brown female pigeon.

(a) Give the genotypes of the parents being mated.

(b) What proportion of the F_1 progeny would be expected to have brown feathers?

(Ans: (a) Male is Bb and the brown female is bb; (b) Half the progeny are expected to have brown feathers.)

1.3.30 Polydactyly, the presence of extra fingers and toes is caused by allele, P, which is dominant to the allele for normal number of digits, p. A man exhibits polydactyly, his father had polydactyly but his mother did not have the abnormality. He marries a normal woman whose family did not have any history of this genetic abnormality.

(a) What are the genotypes of the polydactylous man and the normal woman?

(b) What is the chance/probability of polydactyly in their first child?

(Ans: (a) The person in question is Pp and the normal woman, whom the affected man marries, is pp; (b) The first child could be Pp (polydactylous) or pp (normal). Therefore, the chance (probability) of polydactyly in the first offspring is ½.)

1.3.31 Cystic fibrosis is a serious human disease caused by an allele, c, which is recessive to the allele for the normal condition, C. With appropriate medical care, the persons afflicted with the disease may live to reach early adulthood and beyond. Two phenotypically normal parents have four children: three are normal and one is affected with cystic fibrosis.

(a) Identify the most probable genotypes of the parents.

(b) Identify the most probable genotypes of the children.

(c) What proportion of the normal children is expected to be carrier of the allele responsible for cystic fibrosis?

(Ans: (a) Both the parents are heterozygous, i.e. CcBb; (b) The afflicted child is cc and each of the other three normal children could have either CC or Cc; (c) The proportion of normal children = $\frac{1}{4} + \frac{1}{4} + \frac{1}{4} = \frac{3}{4}$. The proportion of normal children who are carrier = $(\frac{1}{4} + \frac{1}{4})(\frac{3}{4}) = (\frac{1}{2})(\frac{3}{4}) = 2/3$.

1.3.32 In cats, the hairs can be either short or long (referred to as 'angora'). The trait hair length is controlled by a single locus with two alleles. A cat fancier made three different crosses and observed the following results. (1) Angora × angora produced all Angora bunnies. (2) Angora × short produced all short bunnies; and (3) Short × angora produced 4 short and 5 angora bunnies.

(a) Which phenotype is dominant?

(b) What are the genotypes of the parents and offspring for each of the following crosses?

Cross no.	Genotypes of	
	Parents	Bunnies
1	aa × aa	All aa
2	aa × AA	All Aa
3	Aa × aa	½ Aa: ½ aa

(Ans: (a) The allele responsible for short hair is dominant to the allele for angora (long hair). (b) The genotypes for the three crosses would be:

Cross no.	Genotypes of	
	Parents	Bunnies
1	aa × aa	All aa

| 2 | aa × AA | All Aa |
| 3 | Aa × aa | ½ Aa: ½ aa |

1.3.33　In humans, a parent A is feeble-minded and deaf (only one of his parents was deaf), parent B is normal-minded and deaf (only one of her parents was deaf, but one was feeble-minded). N = Normal minded; n = Feeble minded; O = Deaf (Otosclerois) and o = Normal hearing.

(a)　What is the genotypic formula for parent A?

(b)　What is the genotypic formula for parent B?

(c)　Checker-board the possible offspring of A and B.

(d)　What is the ratio of probability that the first child will be: (i) normal-minded, deaf; (ii) normal-minded, hearing; (iii) feeble-minded, deaf; (iv) feeble-minded hearing?

(f)　If six children from these parents fall into the groups of 1, 2 and 3, what is the expectation for the seventh child?

1.3.34　A man with dark, straight hair (DDcc) marries a woman with light, straight hair (ddcc) and they have a son. Another man with light, curly hair (ddCC) marries a woman with dark, straight hair (DDcc) and they have a daughter. The son and daughter marry. Find out their possible offspring and indicate the chance that their first child has the hair, phenotypically (i) like that of the father; (ii) like that of the mother; (iii) unlike that of either.

1.3.35　A child has light, curly hair and dark eyes. The father has light, straight hair and blue eyes. (Light hair, straight hair and blue eyes are recessive). (a) What must have been the phenotype of the mother? (b) What could have been the genotype of the mother?

1.3.36　On an ear of white, sugary corn was found a single kernel of yellow, starchy corn, which showed that this particular kernel had been fertilized by a pollen grain carrying the yellow-starchy character. The embryo for this kernel was therefore hybrid for both yellow and white, as well as for starchy and sugary. The kernel developed into a corn plant and was interbred. The resulting ear bore 465 kernels: 255 yellow-starchy, 91 yellow-sugary, 86 white-starchy and 33 white-sugary.

(a) What would be the expected result? (b) Why there is discrepancy between the actual and expected result?

1.3.37 In sweet peas, the genes P = purple pigment; p = recessive of P; E = actuator of P; e = recessive of E. The possible genotypes and their phenotypes are PePe = white, pEpE = white, PEPE = purple and PepE = purple.

(a) What is the result phenotypically and genotypically when 1 and 2 are crossed?

(b) What is the expectation when the offspring thus produced are self-fertilized?

(c) How many genotypically different white sweet peas are possible from the above formulae? What are they?

(d) How many are genotypically different purple sweet peas? What are they?

(e) What crosses are necessary to produce sweet peas with the genotype of pepE? PEPe?

1.3.38 From the given information on the colours of parents and offspring, figure out the genotypes for each as far as possible. Any dog with B and E is black; with B and no E, red; with E and no B, liver; with neither E nor B, lemon. Each animal is represented by four letters. (a) How many different blacks are possible? (b) What are different kinds of livers and reds? (c) Why are all lemons alike? (d) What are the parental formulae in the following cases?

(a) Liver × red = All black offspring

(b) Liver × red = 1 black, 1 red, 1 liver, 1 lemon

(c) Black × red = 3 black, 1 liver

(d) Black × liver = 3 black, 1 red

(e) Black × liver = 3 black, 3 liver, 1 red, 1 lemon

1.3.39 In pigeons, a dominant allele C causes a checkered pattern in the feathers, its recessive allele c produces a plain pattern. Feather coloration is controlled by an independently assorting gene; the dominant allele B produces red feathers and the recessive allele b produces brown feathers. Birds from a true-breeding checkered, red variety are crossed to birds from a true-breeding plain, brown variety. (a) Predict the phenotype of their progeny, and (b) if these progeny are intercrossed, what phenotypes will appear in the F_2 and in what proportions?

1.3.40 In rabbits, the dominant allele B causes black fur and the recessive allele b causes brown fur; for an independently assorting gene, the dominant allele R causes long fur and the recessive allele r (for *rex*) causes short fur. A homozygous rabbit with long, black fur is crossed with a rabbit with short, brown fur and the offspring are intercrossed. In the F_2, what proportion of the rabbits with long, black fur will be homozygous for both genes?

1.3.41 Albinism in humans is caused by a recessive allele 'a'.

(a) From marriages between people known to be carriers (Aa) and people with albinism (aa), what proportion of the children would be expected to have albinism? Among three children, what is the chance of one with albinism and two without albinism?

(b) If both husband and wife are known to be carriers of the allele for albinism, what is the chance of the following combinations in a family of five children: (i) all five unaffected; (ii) three unaffected and two affected; (c) two unaffected and three affected; (d) one unaffected and four affected?

(c) If a man and a woman are heterozygous for a gene, and if they have four children, what is the chance that all four will also be heterozygous?

1.3.42 Mendel test crossed pea plants grown from yellow, round F_1 seeds to plants grown from green, wrinkled seeds and obtained the results of 30 yellow, round; 35 green, round; 28 yellow, wrinkled; and 27 green, wrinkled. Are these results consistent with the hypothesis that seed colour and seed texture were controlled by independently assorting genes, each segregating two alleles?

1.3.43 The Japanese strain of mice has a peculiar, uncoordinated gait called *waltzing*, which is due to a recessive allele, v. The dominant allele V causes mice to move in a coordinated fashion. A mouse geneticist has recently isolated another recessive mutation that causes uncoordinated movement. This mutation, called *tango*, could be an allele of the waltzing gene, or it could be a mutation in an entirely different gene. Propose a test to determine whether the waltzing and tango mutations are alleles and if they are, propose symbols to denote them.

1.3.44 The summer squash plants with the white fruit (C) are dominant to the plants homozygous for its recessive allele (c) bearing coloured fruit. When the fruit is coloured, the dominant allele G causes it to be yellow; in the absence of this allele (that is, with genotype gg), the fruit colour is green. What are the F_2 phenotypes and proportions expected from intercrossing the progeny of CC GG and cc gg plants? Assume that the C and G genes assort independently.

1.3.45   Fruit flies homozygous for the recessive mutation scarlet have bright red eyes because they cannot synthesize brown pigment. Fruit flies homozygous for the recessive mutation brown have brownish-purple eyes because they cannot synthesize red pigment. Fruit flies homozygous for both of these mutations have white eyes because they cannot synthesize either type of pigment. The brown and scarlet mutations assort independently. If fruit flies that are heterozygous for both of these mutations are intercrossed, what kinds of progeny will they produce, and in what proportions?

1.3.46   A man with dark (dominant), curly hair marries a woman with light, straight hair. They have daughter, who happens to have dark marries a man with light, curly hair. (a) Draw a Punnett's square for this marriage and predict the phenotypic ratio among the offspring of the daughter and her husband. (b) What is the chance that they will have a child with hair just like his or her father's?

1.3.47   In cats, the black colour is dominant to a special, temperature-sensitive albino gene, which produces cats with dark legs, faces and tails. A short-haired (dominant) Siamese coloured female is bred to a long-haired black male. They have eight kittens: 2 black, short haired; 2 black, long haired; 2 Siamese, short haired; and 2 Siamese, long haired. What are the genotypes of the two parents? If pure-breeding (homozygous) black (dominant), long-haired (recessive) cat is mated to a pure-breeding Siamese, short-haired cat, and one of their male offspring is mated to one of their female offspring, what is the chance of producing a Siamese coloured, short-haired kitten?

1.3.48   When a male pig of homozygous black, solid hooved was crossed to a female from homozygous red, cloven-hooved pigs, their progeny all looked alike with regard to colour and hooves. These progeny were all mated to red, cloven-hoofed ones. The offspring from this final cross were 11 black, cloven hooved; 8 black, solid hooved; 14 red, cloven hooved; and 10 red, solid hooved. For each of these two genes (coat colour and hoof type), determine which allele is the dominant one. Explain your reasoning. What were the phenotypes of the progeny produced by the first mating in this problem?

1.3.49 In garden peas, long stems are dominant to short stems and yellow seeds are dominant to green seeds. One hundred long, yellow pea plants, all of which had one short, green parent are interbred (bred to each other), resulting in 1600 progeny. (a) Assuming that these two genes are unlinked, about how many long, green pea plants would you expect to find among the offspring? (b) What ratio of yellow to green seed colour would you expect among the offspring? (c) What would you expect the overall phenotypic ratio among the 1600 offspring to be (taking into consideration both traits)?

1.3.50 In Drosophila, the wild-type eye colour, brick red, is produced by the deposition of two pigments in the eyes, a dull brown pigment and a brilliant red pigment. These two pigments are produced by the action of two different, non-allelic genes. Each of these genes has two alleles: a dominant one which causes normal the production of the pigment, controlled by the gene; and a recessive one, which is defective and causes none of that pigment to be produced. Thus, a normal eye colour fruit fly must have at least one dominant allele for each of these genes.

If a fly is homozygous for the defective, recessive allele of the gene which produces the brown pigment, that fly will have only the brilliant red pigment in its eyes. This condition is called "cinnabar". For this reason, the gene responsible for producing the brown pigment is called the "cinnabar" gene. The symbol for this gene is a two-letter symbol, cn. The dominant allele is Cn and the recessive allele is cn. So, a cinnabar-eyed fly would have the genotype cn cn.

If a fly is homozygous for the defective, recessive allele of the gene, which produces the brilliant red pigment, the fly will have only the dull brown pigment in its eyes. This produces "brown" eyes, so this gene is called the "brown" gene. The symbol for this gene is br. The dominant allele is Br, the recessive br. A brown-eyed fly would be br br.

So, the cinnabar-eyed fly would actually have the genotype cn cn Br Br or cn cn Br br and the brown-eyed fly would have the genotype Cn Cn br br or Cn cn br br.

A mating is made between Cn Cn br br fruit fly and a cn cn Br Br fruit fly, which results into 200 offspring (the F_1). These offspring are allowed to freely interbreed, and produced 40,000 offspring (the F_2),

(a) What colour eyes did the original parents have?

(b) What were the genotypes and phenotypes of the F_1 offspring?

(c) What colour eyes do the cn cn br br flies have?

(d) What phenotypic ratio do you predict among the F_2 offspring?

1.3.51 In humans, cataracts in the eyes and fragility of the bones are caused by dominant alleles that assort independently. A man with cataracts and normal bones marries a woman without cataracts but with fragile bones. The man's father had normal eyes and the woman's father had normal bones. What is the probability that the first child of this couple will (a) be free from both abnormalities, (b) have cataracts but not have fragile bones, (c) have fragile bones but not have cataracts, (d) have both cataracts and fragile bones?

1.3.52 The Drosophila flies homozygous for st have bright red (scarlet) eyes, while St/St and St/st genotypes have the wild-type brick-red eyes. Similarly, the flies homozygous for bw have brown eyes whereas Bw/Bw and Bw/bw genotypes have wild-type brick-red eyes. The double homozygous genotype st/st, bw/bw results in white eyes. In a test of independent assortment of these two genes, a geneticist crossed St/st Bw/bw females to St/st Bw/bw males. Among 480 progeny, there were 300 flies with wild-type eyes, 72 with scarlet eyes, 92 with brown eyes and 16 with white eyes.

(a) If these genes undergo independent assortment, what is the expected numbers in each phenotypic class?

(b) Estimate the Chi-square value.

(Answer: Since this is a dihybrid cross of St/st and Bw/bw × St/st Bw/bw, the ratio of 9:3:3:1 of the offspring phenotypes should be expected if the genes assort independently. We can get the expected number of flies in different classes in progeny generation as:

Phenotype	Genotype	Expected number
Wild type	St/- Bw/-	$(9/16) \times 480 = 270$

Scarlet	st/st Bw/-	$(3/16) \times 480 = 90$
Brown	St/- bw/bw	$(3/16) \times 480 = 90$
White	st/st bw/bw	$(1/16) \times 480 = 30$

The chi-square calculated is 6.76.

1.3.53 A geneticist observed, in a total of 160 individuals, four different phenotypes in the ratio of 91:21:37:11, which he believes that they are in the ratio of 9:3:3:1. Test whether the results agree with the expectation.

1.3.54 Two strains of peas: one with tall vines and violet flowers was crossed with the other with dwarf vines and white flowers. All the F_1 plants were tall and produced violet flowers. When these plants were backcrossed to the dwarf, white parent strain, 53 tall violet, 48 tall white, 47 dwarf violet and 52 dwarf white plants were obtained. Find out whether the genes controlling vine length and flower colour are segregating independently.

1.3.55 In pigeons, a dominant allele C causes a checkered pattern in the feathers; its recessive allele c produces a plain pattern. Feather coloration is controlled by an independently assorting gene, the dominant allele B produces red feathers and its recessive allele b produces brown feathers. Birds from a true breeding checkered, brown variety are crossed to birds from a true breeding plain and red variety.

(a) Predict the phenotype of their progeny.

(b) If these progeny are intercrossed, what phenotypes will appear in the F_2 and in what proportions?

1.3.56 In humans, the dominant autosomal mutation W results in curled hair. Suppose that a woman with curled hair and B-blood group marries a man with straight hair (ww) and AB blood group. The genes are located on different chromosomes.

(a) What are the chances that the marriage will produce curled haired, group-B child?

(b) What are the chances that the marriage will produce straight haired, group-B child?

(c) If three straight-haired children with blood group A are born to these parents, what are the chances that the next child born will be curly-haired and blood group B?

1.4 TRIHYBRID INHERITANCE

A trihybrid cross is between two individuals that are heterozygous for three different traits. We will build on previous examples and again examine pea shape and pea color and then a new trait: pod shape. The same rules as before apply for shape and color (round is completely dominant to wrinkled, and green is completely dominant to yellow). Pea pod shape follows similar rules, with smooth pods being completely dominant to constricted pods. Therefore, homozygous-dominant and heterozygous individuals will have smooth pods, while homozygous-recessive individuals will have constricted pea pods. Our trihybrid cross example:

Table 1.4 Relationship between the number of gene pairs involved in a cross and the number of phenotypes and genotypic classes in F_2.

No. of pairs involved in the cross	No. of different kinds of gametes formed by the F_1 hybrid	No. of genotypically different F_2 combinations	No. of possible combinations in F_2
1	2	3	4
2	4	9	16
3	8	27	64
4	16	81	256
5	32	243	1024
N	2n	3n	4n

The F_2 phenotypic ratio in a trihybrid cross = 27:9:9:9:3:3:3:1

The F_2 genotypic ratio in a trihybrid cross = 1:2:1:2:4:2:1:2:1:2:4:2:4: 8:4:2:4:2:1:2:1:2:4:2:1:2:1

The trihybrid test cross ratio = 1:1:1:1:1:1:1:1

CLASS WORK

1. In garden peas, tall vine (T) is dominant over dwarf (t), green pods over yellow (g), and round seed (R) over wrinkled (r).

    (a) If a homozygous dwarf, green, wrinkled plant is crossed with homozygous tall, yellow and round one, what will be the appearance of the F_1? What gametes does the F_1 form? What will be the appearance of the offspring of a cross of the F_1 with its dwarf, green, wrinkled parent; with its tall, yellow, round parent?

(b) What will be the appearance of the offspring of the following crosses in which the genotypes of the parents are given?

(i) TT Gg Rr × tt Gg rr, (ii) tt gg Rr × Tt Gg rr, (iii) Tt GG Rr × Tt Gg Rr

(c) A tall, green, wrinkled plant crossed with a dwarf, green, round produces offspring three-fourths of which are tall, green, round and one-fourths of which are tall, yellow, round. Find out the genotypes of the parents.

(a)

T = tall	G = green pods	R = round seeds
t = dwarf	g = yellow pods	r = wrinkled seeds

Parents   : dwarf, green, wrinkled × tall, yellow, round

Genotype :   tt GG rr   TT gg RR

Gametes   :   t G r   T g R

F_1 :   Tt Gg Rr

(Tall, green, round)

F_1 gametes :   T G R, t g r   Parental combinations

T g r, t G R   Cross overs between T and g

T G r, t g R   Cross overs between G and r

T g R, t G r   Double crossovers

F_1 × dwarf, green, wrinkled parent

Genotypes :   Tt Gg Rr   ×   tt GG rr

Appearance of the offspring: Ratio:

Tt GG Rr	Tall green round	Tall green round = ¼
tt Gg rr	Dwarf green wrinkled	Tall green wrinkled= ¼
Tt GG rr	Tall green wrinkled	Dwarf green round= ¼
tt GG Rr	Dwarf green wrinkled	Dwarf green wrinkled= ¼
Tt GG rr	Tall green wrinkled	
tt Gg Rr	Dwarf green round	
Tt Gg Rr	Tall green round	
tt GG rr	Dwarf green wrinkled	

F_1 × Tall, yellow, round parent

Genotypes: Tt Gg Rr   ×   Tt gg RR
Appearance of the offspring: Ratio:

Tt Gg Rr	Tall green round	Tall green round = 4/8
Tt gg Rr	Tall yellow round	Tall yellow round = 4/8
TT gg Rr	Tall yellow round	
Tt Gg RR	Tall green round	
TT Gg Rr	Tall green round	
Tt gg RR	Tall yellow round	
Tt gg Rg	Tall yellow round	
Tt Gg Rr	Tall green round	

Since each parent contained a dominant gene for the height, i.e. tall (T) and seed shape, i.e. round (R), all the offspring obtained are tall and round. For the pod colour, one parent is heterozygous green (Gg) and the other homozygous yellow (gg), which forms a test cross, resulted in 1:1 ratio of green and yellow.

HOME WORK

1.4.1   In a cross AaBBCcDdEeFf × AabbccddEeff, what is the probability that an offspring will have genotype AaBbccDdeeFf? (Ans: Probability of Aa Bb cc Dd ee Ff = $\frac{1}{2} \times 1 \times \frac{1}{2} \times \frac{1}{2} \times \frac{1}{4} \times 1$ = 1/32)

1.4.2   The guinea pigs the rosetted (R), short-haired (S) and coloured (C) ones are crossed with smooth (r), long-haired (s) and white guinea pigs; all the offspring appear to be RSC, but the determiners in their germ cells will be RrSsCc. Using the algebraic multiplication, checker-board and bracket methods, find out the answers to: (a) What gametes these trihybrids form? (b) When two such trihybrids are mated, how many and what kinds of offspring will appear genotypically and phenotypically?

1.4.3   In rabbits, the pigmented (P), non-Dutch pattern (D) and short hair (S) are dominant to non-pigmented (p), Dutch pattern (d) and angora (s) hair. What possible genotypes and phenotypes would result if a heterozygous pigmented, pure Dutch pattern, heterozygous short-haired rabbit is crossed with an albino, homozygous non-Dutch pattern, angora rabbit?

1.4.4   In poultry, the white plumage of Leghorns is dominant over the coloured plumage, feathered-shanks over the clean-shanks and pea-comb over the single-comb. When a pure white, feathered, pea-comb bird is crossed with a coloured, clean-shanked, single-combed bird, what proportion of the white feathered, pea-combed birds in F_2 generation in this cross will *breed true* when mated to coloured, clean-shanked, single-combed birds?

1.4.5   In snapdragons, normal regular flowers are dominant over irregular peloric ones and tallness over the dwarfness, while red flower colour is incompletely dominant over white, the heterozygous condition being pink. When a homozygous red, tall, normal-flowered plant is crossed with the nulliplex white, dwarf, peloric-flowered one, what proportion of the F_2 will resemble the F_1 in appearance?

1.4.6   In banana flies, the long-wings (L), red-eyes (W) and gray-body (G) are dominant over the vestigial-wing (l), white-eyes (w) and black-body (b). If the flies of the genotypes LlWwGg are inter-se-mated, how many and what phenotypes are expected? What genotypes are expected?

1.4.7   Suppose that you married a dark-haired individual whose mother was blue-eyed and had a permanent wave; and whose father was bald-headed (recessive) and had a violent temper (dominant). Wavy hair is recessive to curly but dominant to straight. (a) What would be the genotype of your mate? (b) What would be the phenotype of your mate? (c) What is your own phenotype for the characters involved? (d) What is your probable genotype? (e) What would you expect the phenotypic make-up of your first child to be? (f) What would you expect a second child to show?

1.4.8   The peas heterozygous for three independently assorting genes were intercrossed.

    (a) What proportion of the offspring will be homozygous for all three recessive alleles?

    (b) What proportion of the offspring will be homozygous for all the three alleles?

    (c) What proportion of the offspring will be homozygous for one gene and heterozygous for the other two?

    (d) What proportion of the offspring will be homozygous for the recessive allele of at least one gene?

1.4.9   A researcher has discovered a new blood-typing system for human beings. The system involves two antigens: P and Q, each determined by a different allele of a gene named N. The alleles for these antigens are about equally frequent in the general population. If the N and NQ alleles are codominant, what antigens should be detected in the blood of NPNQ heterozygotes? (Ans: Both the P and Q antigens should be detected because codominance implies that both of the alleles will be expressed in the heterozygotes.

1.4.10 In garden peas, tall vine habit (T) is dominant over short vine (t); green pods (G) over yellow (g); and smooth seeds (S) over wrinkled seeds (s). Suppose a homozygous short, green, wrinkled plant is crossed with homozygous tall, yellow, smooth one, what will be the appearance of: (a) F_1? (b) F_2? (c) The offspring of a cross of the F_1 back to its short, green, wrinkled parent? (d) The offspring of a cross of the F_1 back to its tall, yellow, smooth parent?

1.4.11 In a plant breeding experiment, a plant heterozygous for three independently assorting genes, Aa Bb Cc, is self-fertilized. Among the offspring produced, predict the frequency of: (a) AA BB CC plants, (b) aa bb cc plants, (c) plants that are either AA BB CC or aa bb cc, (d) Aa Bb Cc plants and (e) plants that are not heterozygous for all the three genes.

(Answers: a = 1/64; b = 1/64; c = 1/64 + 1/64 = 2/64 = 1/32; d = $\frac{1}{2} \times \frac{1}{2} \times \frac{1}{2}$ = 1/8; e = offspring that are not heterozygous 1 − 1/8 = 7/8)

1.4.12 A plant breeder studied six independently assorting genes in a plant. Each gene has a dominant and recessive allele: R black stem, r red stem; D tall plant, d dwarf plant; C full pods, c constricted pods; O round fruit, o oval fruit; H hairless leaves, h hairy leaves; W purple flower, w white flower. From the cross (P1) rr Dd CC Oo bb Ww × (P2) Rr dd cc oo Hh ww,

(a) How many kinds of gametes can be formed by P1?

(b) How many genotypes are possible among the progeny of this cross?

(c) How many phenotypes are possible among the progeny?

(d) What is the probability of obtaining the Rr Dd Cc Ooh h ww genotype in the progeny?

(e) What is the probability of obtaining a black, dwarf, constricted, oval, hairy, purple phenotype in the progeny?

1.4.13 Based on the given hypothesized situations, determine the degrees of freedom associated with the chi-square statistic and answer whether the observed chi-square value warrants the acceptance or rejection of the hypothesized genetic ratio.

S. no.	Hypothesized genetic ratio	Calculated chi-square value
1	3:1	8.0
2	1:2:1	12.0
3	1:1:1:1	6.0
4	9:3:3:1	2.0

1.4.14 (a) In how many ways can the four gametes A, B, C and D be paired with their respective recessive alleles?

(b) How many different types of gametes are formed by the following parental genotypes: (a) AA, (b) Aa, (c) AaBB, (d) AaBb, (e) AAbbCc, (f) AaBbCcDdEe?

1.4.15 When two plants are crossed, it is found that 63/64 of the progeny are phenotypically like the parents and 1/64 of the progeny are different from either parent but resemble each other. Give the genetic explanation for this.

1.4.16 Assume that a dominant gene causes a pup to grow an additional inch in body height, aabbccddee pups being 12 inches tall. Assume that independent segregation occurs for all gene pairs in the following mating:

AaBBccDdEE × aabbCCDdEe

(a) How tall are the parents?

(b) How tall will the tallest F_1 be?

(c) How tall will the shortest F_1 be?

(d) What proportion of all F_1 will be the shortest?

1.4.17 When the mice of the genotype AaBbCc are mated with another group of same genotype, what proportion of their offspring will be AAbbCc, with an assumption that the three genes segregate independently?

(Choose the correct answer: ½, 1/8, 3/8, 1/32 or 1/64)

1.4.18   How many kinds of gametes can be produced by an individual of the genotype M/m N/n O/o p/p Q/q R/R?

1.4.19 What proportion of the offspring of the cross P/p Q/q R/r × P/p Q/q R/r are expected to be homozygous?

1.4.20   List all the kinds of gametes formed by the following individuals: (a) AABBCc, (b) aaBbCc, (c) AaBbccDd, (d) AABbCcddEeFf

1.4.21   By using '*branching*' technique, find out all possible genotypes of the offspring of the following crosses:
(a) SsYy × SsYy, (b) AaBbCc × AaBbCc, (c) AAbbCcDD × aaBbCcDd

1.4.22   What is the probability that the cross between AaBBCcDd and Aabbccdde will produce the progeny of genotype aaBbCcDd? (Apply multiplication law for individual loci segregations)

1.4.23   A total of six independently assorting genes in a plant were studied. Each gene has a dominant and a recessive allele. R black stem, r red stem; D tall plant, d dwarf plant; C full pods, c constricted pods; O round fruit, o oval fruit; H hairless leaves, h hairy leaves; W purple flower, w white flower. From the cross Rr Dd cc Oo Hh Ww × Rr dd Cc oo Hb ww parents,

(a)   How many kinds of gametes can be formed by P1?

(b)   How many genotypes are possible among the progeny of this cross?

(c)   How many phenotypes are possible among the progeny?

(d)   What is the probability of obtaining the Rr Dd cc Oo hh ww genotype in the progeny?

(e)   What is the probability of obtaining a black, dwarf, constricted, oval, hairy, purple phenotype in the progeny?

PRACTICAL NO. 2

2.1 MODIFIED MONOHYBRID RATIO DUE TO LACK OF DOMINANCE

The lack of dominance or incomplete dominance refers to a genetic situation, in which one allele does not completely dominate another allele, and therefore results in a new (intermediate) phenotype. Such type of inheritance is also known as 'blending inheritance'. Some examples of incomplete dominance are:

- A roan coat colour calf produced by crossing the red-coated and white-coated Shorthorn cattle.
- A black sheep and a white sheep mate and have a grey sheep.
- A long-tailed dog and a short-tailed dog mated, and the offspring has a medium lengthened tail.
- A snapdragon flower that is pink as a result of cross-pollination between a red flower and a white flower, when neither white nor the red alleles are dominant.
- An Andalusian fowl produced from a black and a white parent is blue.
- A brown fur coat on a rabbit as a result of one rabbit's red allele and one rabbit's white allele not dominating.
- A short-haired dog and a long-haired dog mate and the resulting offspring have medium length hair.
- Sickle cell disease is the result of incomplete dominance as those who have the disease carry 50% normal and 50% abnormal hemoglobin.

The modified F_2 phenotypic ratio due to lack of dominance = 1:2:1

CLASS WORK

1. In Shorthorn cattle, the gene for red coat colour (R) is incompletely dominant over the gene for white (r). The heterozygotes of red and white (Rr) result in roan colour. If a homozygous red bull is crossed to a white cow, what will be the appearance of F_1 and F_2? Of the offspring of a cross of F_1 with red parent and with white parent?

Phenotype:	Red	×	white	
Genotype:	RR	×	rr	
Gametes formed:	R	R	r	r

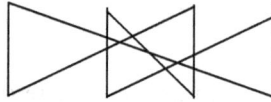

F$_1$ offspring:	Rr	Rr	Rr	Rr
		All roan calves		
F$_2$	roan	×	roan	
	Rr	×	Rr	
Gametes formed:	R	r	R	r

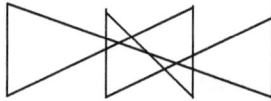

F$_2$ offspring:	RR	rr	Rr	Rr
	Red	white	roan	roan

F$_2$ phenotypic ratio :   1 Red   :   2 roan   :   1 white
F$_2$ genotypic ratio: 1 RR   :   2 Rr   :   1 rr

It may be observed that the F$_2$ phenotypic and genotypic ratios are same.

Cross of F$_1$ offspring with red parent:

Phenotype:	roan	×	Red	
Genotype:	Rr	×	RR	
Gametes formed:	R	r	R	R

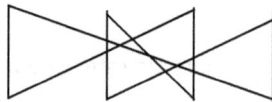

Offspring:	RR	Rr	Rr	RR
Phenotype:	Red	roan	roan	red

Phenotypic ratio: Red : roan = 1 : 1

Cross of F$_1$ offspring with white parent:

Phenotype:	roan	×	white
Genotype:	Rr	×	rr

Gametes formed: R   r   r   r

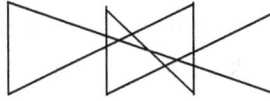

Offspring: Rr   rr   rr   Rr
Phenotype: roan   white   white   roan
Phenotypic ratio: roan : white = 1 : 1

Some of the typical examples for incomplete dominance/co-dominance are:

1. Coat colour in Shorthorn cattle:
   RR = Red; Rr = roan; rr = white
2. Feather colour in poultry (Andalusian fowls)
   BB = Black; Bb = blue; bb = white
3. Feather structure
   NN = normal; NW = frizzled; WW = woolly
4. Naked neck in poultry
   Na Na = naked neck; Na na = naked neck with tuft of feathers; na na = normal neck
5. Coat colour in horses
   CC = chestnut (reddish); c^{cr} c^{cr} = cremello (whitish); Cc^{cr} = palomino pattern i.e., golden or yellow body with white mane and tail
6. MN blood groups in humans
   MM = M blood group; MN = MN blood group; NN = N blood group
7. Hair structure in humans
   A_1A_1 = straight hair; A_1A_2 = wavy hair; A_2A_2 = curly hair
8. Hemoglobin type in humans
   Hb^A Hb^A = Type A; Hb^S Hb^S = Type S; Hb^A Hb^S = Type AS

HOME WORK

2.1.1   Coat colour in guinea pigs is governed by a pair of codominant alleles: C^Y and C^W such that C^YC^Y are yellow; C^YC^W are cream and

C^WC^W are white. If the cream-coated males are mated to yellow-coated females and the resulting F_1 are allowed to mate among them, what phenotypic ratio/proportion is expected in the F_2?

2.1.2   In four-O'clock plants, red (R) flower colour is incompletely dominant over white (r) and F_1 produces pink flowers. A plant with pink flowers was self-pollinated and also crossed with one having red flowers and other white flowers. Find out the genoytpes and phenotypes of the parents and their offspring.

2.1.3   In Shorthorn cattle, the genotype RR causes a red coat, the genotype rr causes a white coat and the genotype Rr causes a roan coat. A breeder has red, white and roan cows and bulls. What phenotypes may be expected from the following matings and in what proportions?

(a) red × roan, (b) red × red, (c) roan × roan, (d) white × roan, (e) red × white

2.1.4   In humans, the gene for curly hair (C) is incompletely dominant over the straight (c) such that the heterozygotes (Cc) have the wavy hair. Two-way haired people (one male and one female) marry and have eight children. Of these eight, how many would you expect to be curly haired? How many wavy haired and how many straight haired, assuming that the family follows the expected statistically predicted pattern? Suppose you examine the actual children and discover that three of the eight have curly hair, what do you suppose went wrong?

2.1.5   The body colour in horses is influenced by several genes. Two of these alleles, the chestnut (dark brown) and a diluting (pale cream) alleles display incomplete dominance. A horse heterozygous for these two alleles is a palomino (golden body colour with flaxen mane and tail). Is it possible to produce a herd of pure breeding palomino horses? Why or why not? Work out the Punnett's square for mating a palomino to a palomino and predict the phenotypic ratio among their offspring.

2.1.6   In human beings, there is a genetic disease called *Tay Sachs* disease, which is caused by a recessive allele of a single gene, is fatal to infants within the first 5 years of life. Why does this disease persist, even though it is invariably fatal long before the afflicted individual reaches the reproductive age? In other words, explain why the allele for *Tay Sachs* disease simply doesn't disappear.

2.1.7   If an allele R is dominant over the allele r, how many different phenotypes are expected to be present in the progeny of a cross between Rr and Rr and in what ratio? If there is no dominance between R and r, how many phenotypes and in what ratio would be present in the offspring of the cross: Rr × Rr?

2.1.8   In cattle black coat colour is dominant (B) over red (b), while red (R) and white give roan (r).

(a) Explain how a pure hereditary trait may be derived from two parents who are impure for the trait in question.

(b) What is the expectation in the following crosses?
    (i) Homozygous black × homozygous black
    (ii) Homozygous black × heterozygous black
    (iii) Homozygous black × red
    (iv) Heterozygous black × heterozygous black
    (v) Heterozygous black × red
    (vi) Red × red
    (vii) Red × roan
    (viii) Roan × white
    (ix) Roan × roan
    (x) White × white

2.1.9   In Shorthorn cattle, the polled (P) condition is dominant over horned (p), and roan is the result of the heterozygous condition of genes for red (R) and white (r). What proportion of the offspring of a roan heterozygous polled bull and roan horned cow would be expected to be roan and horned?

2.1.10   In cattle, the hornless or polled condition (P) is dominant over horned (p); and the hybrid from red-coat (R) and white-coat (r) is roan.

(a) What will be the appearance of the offspring from a pure polled white and pure horned red animal?

(b) What will be the result if this offspring is crossed back to the white parent?

(c) What will be the result if the same offspring is crossed with the red parent?

(d) A polled, roan bull bred to a white, horned cow produces a roan heifer. What may be the offspring from this heifer bred back to her father, as to colour and condition of horns?

2.2 MODIFIED DIHYBRID RATIO DUE TO LACK OF DOMINANCE IN ONE PAIR

The classical F_2 ratio in dihybrid inheritance is modified due to lack of dominance in one of the two pairs of genes, and this result in more than four phenotypes in F_2 generation. The modified dihybrid ratio (F_2) due to lack of dominance in one pair of genes is 3:6:3:1:2:1.

CLASS WORK

1. In cattle, polled condition (P) is dominant over horned (p), and in Shorthorns the heterozygous condition of red (R) and white (r) coat is roan.

    (a) If a homozygous polled, white animal is bred to a horned red one, what will be the appearance of F_1 and F_2? What will be the genotypic ratio in F_2? What will be the appearance of the offspring of a cross of F_1 with the polled white parent and with the horned red parent?

    (b) What proportion of the offspring of a roan heterozygous polled bull and roan horned cow would be expected to be roan and horned?

    (c) A polled roan bull bred to a horned white cow, produces a horned roan calf. If this calf is bred to its sire, what offspring may be expected with regard to horns and coat colour?

(a) Parents: Polled white   ×   horned red

    Genotype: PPrr   ppRR

    F_1 Polled roan

                                    PpRr

    F_2 PpRr   ×   PpRr

    Gametes: PR Pr pR pr   ×   PR Pr pR pr

The phenotypes and genotypes obtained in F_2 generation can be shown in the form of checker-board as:

F_2 Offspring:

♂ ♀	PR	Pr	pR	pr
PR	PPRR (Polled Red)	PPRr (Polled Roan)	PpRR (Polled Red)	PpRr (Polled Roan)
Pr	PPRr (Polled Roan)	PPrr (Polled White)	PpRr (Polled Roan)	Pprr (Polled White)
pR	PpRR (Polled Red)	PpRr (Polled Roan)	ppRR (Horned Red)	ppRr (Horned Roan)
pr	PpRr (Polled Roan)	Pprr (Polled White)	ppRr (Horned Roan)	Pprr (Horned White)

F_2 phenotypic ratio:

Polled, Red	:	3	Horned, Red	:	1
Polled, Roan	:	6	Horned, Roan	:	2
Polled, White	:	3	Horned, White	:	1

The F_2 genotypic ratio is:

Segregation at first locus (Polled vs. horned)		Segregation at second locus (Red vs. white coat)	Simultaneous segregation for the two loci
¼ PP	×	¼ RR	1/16 PPRR
¼ PP	×	½ Rr	2/16 PPRr
¼ PP	×	¼ rr	1/16 PPrr
½ Pp	×	¼ RR	2/16 PpRR
½ Pp	×	½ Rr	4/16 PpRr
½ Pp	×	¼ rr	2/16 Pprr
¼ pp	×	¼ RR	1/16 ppRR
¼ pp	×	½ Rr	2/16 ppRr
¼ pp	×	¼ rr	1/16 pprr

Therefore, the F_2 genotypic ratio observed is 1:2:1:2:4:2:1:2:1

F_1 × Polled white parent:

Genotype	:	PpRr	×	PPrr	
Gametes	:	PR Pr pR pr	Pr	
Offspring	:				

♂ ♀	PR	Pr	pR	pr
Pr	PPRr (Polled, roan)	PPrr (Polled, white)	PpRr (Polled, roan)	Pprr (Polled, white)

Polled roan: polled white = 1:1

F_1 × horned red parent:

Genotype   :   PpRr   ×   ppRR

Gametes   :   PR   Pr   pR   pr   pR

Offspring   :

♂ ♀	PR	Pr	pR	pr
pR	PpRR (Polled red)	PpRr (Polled roan)	ppRR (Horned red)	ppRr (Horned roan)

Polled red: Polled roan: Horned red: Horned roan= 1:1:1:1

(b) Parents   :   Polled roan   ×   Horned roan

Genotype   :   PpRr   ×   ppRr

Gametes   :   PR   Pr   pR   pr   pR   pr

Offspring   :

♂ ♀	PR	Pr	pR	pr
pR	PpRR (Polled red)	PpRr (Polled roan)	ppRR (Horned red)	ppRr (Horned roan)
pr	PpRr (Polled roan)	Pprr (Polled white)	ppRr (Horned roan)	pprr (Horned white)

Proportion of horned roan offspring = 2/8 or 25%

(c) Parents   :   Polled roan bull   ×   Horned white cow

Genotype   :   PpRr   ×   pprr

Phenotype of F_1 :   Horned roan

(ppRr)

F_1 offspring   ×   Polled roan male parent

Gametes   : pR   pr   ×   PR   Pr   pR   pr

Offspring   :

♂ ⁄ ♀	PR	Pr	pR	pr
pR	PpRR (Polled red)	PpRr (Polled roan)	ppRR (Horned red)	ppRr (Horned roan)
pr	PpRr (Polled roan)	Pprr (Polled white)	ppRr (Horned roan)	pprr (Horned white)

Polled red	:	1	Horned red	:	1
Polled roan	:	2	Horned roan	:	2
Polled white	:	1	Horned white	:	1

HOME WORK

2.2.1   In peaches, fuzzy skin (F) is completely dominant over smooth skin (f), and the heterozygous condition of oval glands at the base of the leaves (O) and no glands (o) gives round glands. A homozygous fuzzy, no-gland peach variety is bred to a smooth, oval-gland variety.

(a) What will be the appearance of the F_1 and F_2?

(b) What will be the appearance of the offspring of a cross of the F_1 back to the smooth, oval-glanded parent?

2.2.2   The coat in guinea pigs may be either long or short; matings of short × short may produce long-haired progeny, but long × long gives rise only to long. Additionally, coat colour may be yellow, cream or white. The mating cream × cream produces progeny of each of the three colours. When the following incomplete pedigree is given,

P: Long yellow × short white

F_1: All short,

(a) What will be the coat colour in F_1?

(b) If members of the F_1 were interbred, what fraction of their progeny would be long cream?

2.2.3   Feather colour in chickens is governed by a single locus involving codominant alleles: B = black, W = white, such as BB are black, BW are blue and WW are white plumage colour. A second locus, carried on a different pair of chromosomes, controls the presence or absence of feathers on the legs. The dominant allele F produces feathered legs, while its recessive counterpart f produces featherless legs. A black cock with feathered legs and derived from pure-breeding stock mates with a white hen with featherless legs.

(a) What would be the genotypes and phenotypes of the F_1 progeny produced from this mating?

(b) If the F_1 chickens are allowed to mate among themselves, give the phenotypes of their offspring and the frequencies with which each phenotypic class is expected to occur.

(c) Assume that an F_2 blue chicken with featherless legs of genotype BWff is backcrossed with its mother of genotype BWFf. Calculate the probability of obtaining (i) an offspring of blue colour with featherless legs and (ii) an offspring of white colour with feathered legs?

2.2.4   A dominant allele L governs short hair in guinea pigs and its recessive allele l causes long hair. Codominant alleles at an independently assorting locus specify hair colour, such that $C^Y C^Y$ = yellow, $C^Y C^W$ = cream and $C^W C^W$ = white. From matings between dihybrid short, cream pigs (Ll $C^Y C^W$), predict the phenotypic ratio expected in the progeny.

2.2.5   In cattle, the allele for absence of horns or polled (H) is completely dominant over the horned (p) so that HH and Hh are hornless or polled and hh is horned. In contrast, the allele producing red coat colour (R) is incompletely dominant over the white (r). The heterozygous genotype Rr is roan coloured, which is an intermediate colour in which the white hair are intermixed with red ones. The alleles H and R segregate and assort independent of each other.

(a) What would be the phenotype of the offspring (F_1) resulting from the mating of the parents with genotypes RR HH and rr hh?

(b) What would be the phenotypes and their expected proportions in F_2 progeny of the cross $F_1 \times F_1$ from part (a)?

(c) What would be the phenotypes and their expected proportions among the progeny derived from crossing F_1 individuals from part (a) to the original horned white stock?

2.3 MODIFIED DIHYBRID RATIO DUE TO LACK OF DOMINANCE IN BOTH PAIRS

The classical F_2 dihybrid ratio is modified due to lack of dominance in both the pairs of genes, and it results in nine different phenotypes. The F_2 phenotypic as well as genotypic ratio is modified into 1:2:1:2:4:2:1:2:1.

CLASS WORK

1. In Snapdragon, red flower colour (R) is incompletely dominant over white (r) with the heterozygotes expressed as pink. Broad leaves (B) are incompletely dominant over narrow (b), the heterozygotes being intermediate leaf breadth. If a red-flowered, broad-leaved plant is crossed with a white-flowered narrow-leaved one, what will be the appearance of F_1 and F_2?

Flower colour: Leaf size:

    RR = Red   BB = Broad

    Rr = Pink   Bb = Intermediate

    rr = White   bb = narrow

Parents   :   Red broad   ×   Narrow white

Genotypes   :   RRBB   ×   rrbb

F_1 offspring   :   RrBb

                      (All pink, intermediate)

F_2 :   RrBb   ×   RrBb

F_2 offspring:

♀ \ ♂	RB	Rb	rB	rb
RB	RRBB (Red broad)	RRBb (Red intermediate)	RrBB (Pink broad)	RrBb (Pink intermediate)
Rb	RRBb (Red intermediate)	RRbb (Red narrow)	RrBb (Pink intermediate)	Rrbb (Pink narrow)
rB	RrBB (Pink broad)	RrBb (Pink intermediate)	rrBB (White broad)	rrBb (White intermediate)
rb	RrBb (Pink intermediate)	Rrbb (Pink narrow)	rrBb (White intermediate)	rrbb (White narrow)

F_2 phenotypic ratio:

Red broad	: 1	Pink broad	: 2	White broad	: 1
Red intermediate	: 2	Pink intermediate	: 4	White intermediate	: 2
Red narrow	: 1	Pink white	: 2	White narrow	: 1

HOME WORK

2.3.1   In Snapdragon, red flower colour (R) is incompletely dominant over white (r). Broad leaves (B) are incompletely dominant over narrow (b). What will be the genotypes and phenotypes and in what proportion of F_2 of a cross between red broad and white narrow?

2.3.2   Feather colour in chickens is governed by a single locus involving codominant alleles; FB and FW such that FBFB are black, FBFW are blue and FWFW are white (the symbols B and W are used for black and white, respectively). Feather shape/morphology is governed by another locus with codominant alleles such that MNMN = normal shape, MNMF = mildly abnormal (mild frizzled) and MFMF = grossly abnormal (called extreme frizzled; symbols N and F are used for the two alleles). If blue, mildly frizzled birds are crossed among themselves, what phenotypic proportions/ratios are expected among their offspring? (Ans: 1:2:1:2:4:2:1:2:1)

2.3.3   The shape and colour of radishes are controlled by two independent pairs of alleles that show no dominance; each genotype is distinguishable phenotypically. The colour may be red (RR), purple (Rr) or white (rr) and the shape may be long (LL), oval (Ll) or round (ll). Depict diagrammatically, the cross between red, long (RRLL) and white, round (rrll) radishes, and summarize the F_2 progeny under the headings: phenotypes, genotypes, genotypic and phenotypic ratios.

2.3.4   Seven colours are produced in the Four-O'clock (*Mirabilis*) plant by two factors and their allelomorphs as detailed: crimson (YYRR), orange-red (YYRr), yellow (YYrr), magenta (YyRR), magenta-rose (YyRr), pale yellow (Yyrr) and white (yyRR) and (yyrr).

(a) Which parental Four-O'clocks are capable of producing every colour named except yellow and pale yellow?

(b) What parents will produce pale yellow?

2.3.5   About 100 tomato plants from some unknown seed were raised and found 37 red fruited with scattered short hairs on stems and leaves, 19 red hairless, 18 red very hairy, 13 yellow-fruited with scattered short hairs, 7 yellow very hairy and 6 yellow hairless. Suggest the genotypes and phenotypes for the unknown parent plants from which the 100 seeds were obtained.

2.3.6   The colour of feathers in chickens is influenced by a pair of codominant alleles in such a way that the genotype F^BF^B produces black, F^WF^W produces splashed white and F^BF^W causes blue colour. An independently segregating locus influences length of leg. Genotypes CC have normal leg length, CC^L produces squatty, short-legged types called *creepers*, but the homozygous C^LC^L genotypes are lethal. Determine the kinds of progeny phenotypes and their expected ratios in the crosses between dihybrid blue creepers are likely to produce.

PRACTICAL NO. 3

3.1 GENE INTERACTION

The Mendelian ratios of 3:1 and 9:3:3:1 do not occur in all crosses since many characters are influenced by two or more pairs of genes and the expressions of these genes interact. Depending upon the form of interaction, the phenotypic ratios are modified in various ways although the fundamental laws of transmission of heredity remain the same.

CLASS WORK

A classical case of two genes influencing the same trait as discovered by Bateson and Punnett in fowls is explained below.

The Wyandotte breed has a comb known as *rose comb*; Brahmas have *pea comb* and Leghorns have *single comb*. In crosses between rose combed and single combed, the rose was dominant over single; and in crosses between the pea and single combed birds, pea was dominant over single. When rose was crossed with the pea, the F_1 hybrids showed new forms of combs known as *walnut* and *single*.

Parents	:	Rose	×	Pea
Genotypes	:	RRpp		rrPP
Gametes	:	Rp		rP
F_1	:		RrPp	
		All Walnut combed		
F_2	:	RrPp	×	RrPp
Gametes	:	RP Rp rP rp		RP Rp rP rp
F_2 offspring	:			

♂ / ♀	RP	Rp	rP	rp
RP	RRPP (Walnut)	RRPp (Walnut)	RrPP (Walnut)	RrPp (Walnut)
Rp	RRPp (Walnut)	RRpp (Rose)	RrPp (Walnut)	Rrpp (Rose)

rP	RrPP	RrPp	rrPP	rrPp
	(Walnut)	(Walnut)	(Pea)	(Pea)
rp	RRPp	RRpp	RrPp	rrpp
	(Walnut)	(Rose)	(Walnut)	(Single)

F_2 phenotypic ratio = 9 walnut: 3 rose: 3 pea: 1 single

HOME WORK

3.1.1   In poultry, the genes for rose comb (R) and pea comb (P) together produce walnut comb. The alleles of both in homozygous recessive condition (rrpp) produce single comb. From information concerning interactions of these genes given in the class, determine the phenotypes and proportions expected from the following crosses.

(a) RRPp × rrPp, (b) rrPP × RrPp, (c) RrPp × Rrpp, (d) Rrpp × rrpp, (e) Rrpp × Rrpp

3.1.2   For the following crosses involving the comb characters in poultry, determine the genotypes of the two parents:

(a) A walnut crossed with a single produces offspring, ¼ of which are walnut, ¼ rose, ¼ pea and ¼ single.

(b) A rose crossed with a walnut produces offspring, 3/8 of which are walnut, 3/8 rose, 1/8 pea and 1/8 single.

(c) A rose crossed with a pea produces 5 walnut and 6 rose offspring.

(d) A walnut crossed with a walnut produces 1 rose, 2 walnuts and 1 single offspring.

(e) Walnut × pea combed cross produced 15 walnut-, 14 rose-, 5 pea- and 6 single-combed individuals.

(f) A rose crossed with another rose produced 3/4 rose and 1/4 pea, 1/4 walnut and 1/4 single combed.

(g) A homozygous walnut-combed bird crossed with a single combed. Determine the comb types appearing in F_1 and F_2.

(h) A walnut-combed fowl mated with a rose produced all walnut-combed progenies.

(i) Two walnut-combed chickens are mated to each other and produce walnut- and rose-combed offspring in the ratio of 3:1. What are the genotypes of the parents?

(j) Rose-combed chickens mated with walnut-combed chickens produced 20 walnut-, 10 rose-, 4 pea- and 8 single-combed chicks. Determine the genotypes of the parents.

3.1.3   The presence of feathers on the legs of chickens is due to a dominant allele (F) and clean legs to its recessive allele (f). Pea-combed shape is produced by another dominant allele (P) and single comb by its recessive allele (p). In crosses between pure-feathered leg, single-combed individuals and pure pea-combed, clean leg individuals, suppose that only single-combed, feathered leg F_2 progeny are saved and allowed to mate at random. What genotypic and phenotypic ratios would be expected among the progeny (F_3)?

3.1.4   Large number of birds with all the four kinds of comb, i.e. walnut, rose, pea and single, were available in a farm. If the breeding operations were started by crossing the pea-combed and rose-combed fowls, what matings would you perform to obtain a pure-breeding single-combed stock?

3.1.5   In poultry, feathered shanks (F) are dominant over clean (f). A feather-shanked, rose-combed bird crossed with a clean-shanked, pea-combed one produces 25 feathered, pea offspring; 24 feathered, walnut; 26 feathered, rose; and 22 feathered, single. Find out the genotypes of the parents.

3.1.6   Red kernel colour in wheat results from the presence of at least one dominant allele at each of two independently segregating genes, i.e. R-B-. Kernels on doubly homozygous recessive plants are white and the genotypes R_bb and rrB_ result in brown kernel colour. If plants of a variety that is true breeding for red kernels are crossed with plants true breeding for white kernels, (a) what is the expected phenotype of the F_1 plants? (b) What are the expected phenotypic classes and their relative proportions in the F_2 progeny?

3.1.7   In fowls, the genes for rose (R) and pea (P) if present together result in walnut comb (R_P_). The recessive alleles of both in homozygous form produce single comb. What will be the comb appearance in the offspring of the following crosses?

(a) RrPp × RrPp   (b) RrPp × rrPp   (c) RrPp × Rrpp
(d) RrPp × rrpp   (e) Rrpp × RrPP   (f) RRpp × rrpp
(g) RRPP × rrpp

3.1.8 A poultry farmer has started breeding with pure-breeding stocks of pea- and rose-combed fowls. What phenotypic ratio is expected in the offspring if a dihybrid individual for comb shape is test crossed? What matings would he required for a true breeding single combed stock?

3.1.9 In mice, the brown agouti mice are called "*cinnamons*". When wild-type mice are crossed with cinnamons, the $F_1(s)$ are all wild type and the F_2 consists of three wild type and one cinnamon. (a) Diagram this cross by taking B = black of the wild type, b = brown of the cinnamon. In the F_2, besides the parental type (cinnamon and non-agouti strain of black) and the wild type of the F_1, a fourth colour called *chocolate* shows up. Chocolates are a solid, rich brown colour. What do the chocolates represent genetically? What phenotypes and in what proportions would be observed in the progeny of a backcross of the $F_1(s)$ to the cinnamon parent stock? To the non-agouti (black) parent stock? Diagram these backcrosses. If a test cross is conducted, what colours would result and in what proportions?

3.1.10 In poultry, there are four homozygous phenotypes with respect to combs – rose (RRpp), pea (rrPP), walnut (RRPP) and single (rrpp).
(a) Starting with a rose and pea how is it possible to get the other two kinds?
(b) How many are genotypically different walnut combs? What are they?
(c) What kind of a walnut comb would be required to produce all four types of combs when crossed with a single comb?

3.1.11 In Drosophila, the recessive gene *sable* (x) causes a black body colour. Another gene, the *recessive suppressor of sable* (t) prevents expression of the sable gene, so the fly is normal gray colour. Thus, the genotypes s/s T/- are sable, all others are normal (s/s t/t, S/-T/-, S/-t/t). What offspring would be expected from the cross S/s T/t × s/s T/t?

3.1.12 In humans, the gene D is essential for a normal ear cochlea and gene E is necessary for a normal auditory nerve. In the absence of either of these factors, the individual is deaf. Show how two normal parents could produce a deaf child and how two deaf parents could produce a normal child.

3.1.13   In rice, *awned* condition is due to the presence of genes A or B or both and *awnless* is due to the presence of both recessive genes (aa bb). What will be the appearance of F_1 and F_2 progenies from a cross between homozygous awned and awnless? Give the genotype of the parents.

3.1.14   In Drosophila, recessive mutations in either of two independently assorting genes, brown and purple, prevent the synthesis of red pigment in the eyes. Thus, homozygotes for either of these mutations have brownish-purple eyes. However, heterozygotes for both of these mutations have dark red, that is, wild-type eyes. If such double heterozygotes are intercrossed, what kinds of progeny will be produced and in what proportions?

3.1.15   The Drosophila flies homozygous for the recessive mutation *scarlet* have bright red eyes because they cannot synthesize brown pigment. Fruit flies homozygous for the recessive mutation *brown* have brownish-purple eyes because they cannot synthesize red pigment. The flies homozygous for both of these mutations have white eyes because they cannot synthesize either type of pigment. The *brown* and *scarlet* mutations assort independently. If a fly heterozygous for both of these mutations is crossed with a fly that is homozygous recessive for both of these mutations, what kinds of progeny will they produce and in what proportions?

3.2 EPISTASIS

Epistasis is defined as the interaction between the non-allelic genes. Epistasis is the best example for gene interaction. It is a pattern of inheritance where a pair of genes situated at one locus, prevent the expression of a pair of genes situated at another locus. Such genes are called inhibiting genes or epistatic genes (Epi = above/over gene, static = standing). It is an intergenic or non-allelic form of gene interaction. The basic genes, the expression of which is prevented by the epistatic genes, are called as hypostatic genes. Epistasis reduces the number of phenotypes in the F_2 generation of a dihybrid cross. The gene which blocks the expression is called *epistatic*, while the one whose expression is blocked is called *hypostatic*.

A classical example of epistasis is seen in the white fowls. There are two varieties of white fowls: white Leghorn and white Plymouth Rock. A cross between a homozygous dominant, white Leghorn and homozygous recessive white Plymouth Rock results in a progeny of F_1 generation containing dihybrid white progeny and of the F_2 generation consists of white and coloured fowls in the ratio of 13:3 in place of the normal phenotypic ratio of 9:3:3:1. In addition, there is a reduction in the number of phenotypes to just two.

The basic gene C produces colour in the feathers. But the inhibiting gene I prevents the appearance of colour. Gene I interacts with gene C in such a way to suppress its expression. As a result the Leghorn fowl is white CCII. The Plymouth Rock fowl is white since it has recessive genes ccii. In the F_1 generation all the progeny are white but heterozygous (CcIi), when these fowls are allowed to inbreed, in the F_2 generation, the genotypes having gene I along with gene C will produce white fowls. The genotypes which do not have gene I give rise to coloured fowls.

Plumage colour in chickens is determined by several loci. But, here we shall consider only the interaction between C locus and I locus.

C locus dominant allele allows melanin production.

c prevents the melanin production.

Therefore, CC = coloured; Cc = coloured; cc = homozygous recessives are white as no colour is produced.

I locus:

I = dominant allele inhibits the action of feather colour gene, C; i.e., I is epistatic to C gene. Thus, the genotypes and their phenotypes are:

Genotypes	Genotypic notation	Phenotype
CCII; CCIi CcIi; CcII ccII; ccIi; ccii	C_I_ CcI_ cc _ _	White
CC; Ccii	C_ii	Colored

P₁   Phenotype: White Leghorn Fowl × Plymouth Rock Fowl
Genotype: CCII   ccii
Gametes: CI   ci
F_1 genotype   CcIi
F_1 phenotype   Heterozygous white Leghorn
F_1 gametes   CI   Ci   cI   ci
F_2 offspring:

	CI	Ci	cI	ci
CI	CCII White	CCIi White	CcII White	CCIi White
Ci	CCIi White	CCii Coloured	CcIi White	CCii Colored
cI	CcII White	CcIi White	ccII White	CcIi White
ci	CCIi White	CCii Coloured	CcIi White	ccii White

Therefore, modified dihybrid ratio due to epistasis is 13:3 white:coloured fowl.

The examples for different epistasis ratios are:

F_2 phenotype	F_2 phenotypic ratio
Coat colour in mouse	9:3:4 black: white: albino
Fruit colour in squash	12:3:1 white, yellow, green
Flower colour in peas	9:7 purple: white
Fruit shape in squash	9:6:1 disc: circular: long
Fruit shape in shepherds purse	15:1 triangular: ovoid
Feather colour in fowls	13:3 white: coloured

The coat colour in Labrador dogs is an example for epistasis. The Labradors have 3 basic recognised coat colours namely, black, brown (or chocolate) and yellow (Golden). Two loci, B and E determine the above colours.

B = black; b = brown; E = extension of pigment locus. The E gene allows the extension of black or brown pigment to the hairs, while e gene in homozygous state does not permit extension of black or brown pigment to the hairs. Hence, coat appears as yellow or golden.

Therefore, the genotype B_E_ (BBEE, BBEe, BbEE and BbEe) causes black; bbE_ (bbEE, bbEe) causes brown while _ _ ee (BBee, Bbee and bbee) causes golden yellow.

Parents phenotypes   :   Yellow   ×   Brown
Parents genotypes   :   BBee   ×   bbEE
F_1 BbEe (Black)
F_2 offspring   :

	BE	Be	bE	be
BE	BBEE Black	BBEe Black	BbEE Black	BbEe Black
Be	BBEe Black	BBee Yellow	BbEe Black	Bbee Yellow
bE	BbEE Black	BbEe Black	bbEE Brown	bbEe Brown
be	BbEe Black	Bbee Yellow	bbEe Brown	bbee yellow

Thus, modified Mendelian ratio due to recessive epistasis is 9 Black: 3 Brown: 4 yellow.

HOME WORK

3.2.1   White Leghorn chickens are known to be homozygous for a dominant allele C of a gene responsible for coloured feathers and also for a dominant allele I that prevents the expression of C. The white Wyandotte breed is homozygous recessive for both the genes. What proportion of the F_2 progeny from white Leghorn × white Wyandotte F_1 hybrids can be expected to have coloured feathers?

3.2.2   In mice, the genotype C_ is responsible for pigmented skin, while the individuals of cc genotype are albinos. Another pair of genotypes B_ and bb results in black and brown coat, respectively. What will be the appearance of F_2 offspring of a cross of CCBB × ccbb?

3.2.3   In the F_2 from a particular cross, a modified dihybrid ratio of 9:7 is obtained. What corresponding ratio would you expect from a test cross of the F_1s?

3.2.4   In mice, black coat colour is due to a dominant gene C; albino is due to its recessive allele c in homozygous condition. Another gene A has no phenotypic effect of its own but when present in addition to C modifies black coat colour into agouti. Two agouti mice are mated. Among the progenies of this cross 9/16 are agouti, 3/16 are black and 4/16 are albino. Find the genotypes of the parents and genetic mechanism involved.

3.2.5   A cross between two green plants of maize produced offspring of which about 9/16 were green and 7/16 were white. Explain these results genetically.

3.2.6   In chickens, the genotype C/- O/- i/i is coloured, all other combinations being white. Leghorns are C/C O/O I/I, white Wyandottes are c/c O/O i/I and white Silkies are C/C o/o i/i. What offspring would be expected from the following?
(a) A white Silkie crossed with a white Wyandotte?
(b) A white Leghorn crossed with a white Silkie?
(c) A Leghorn–Silkie hybrid backcrossed to a Silkie?
(d) A Leghorn–Silkie hybrid crossed with a Wyandotte?

3.2.7   In squashes, white fruit colour is dependent on a dominant gene W and coloured on its recessive gene w. In the presence of G and ww fruit colour is yellow, but when G is not present, i.e. gg, the colour is green.
(a) What will be phenotypes of the offspring resulting from the following crosses?
      (i) wwGG × Wwgg, (ii) Wwgg × wwGg, (iii) WwGg × WwGg, (iv) WWgg × wwGG
(b) A white-fruited plant (WWGG) of summer squash is crossed with a green-fruited plant (wwgg). What phenotypic frequencies are expected in F_2 generation?

(c) A cross of white squash plant with yellow gave the progenies in the ratio of ½ white, 3/8 yellow and 1/8 green. Determine the genotype of the parents and offspring.

(d) A cross between white and green squash plant produces 50 white and 50 yellow offspring. Give the genotype of the parents.

(e) A cross of white squash with another one gave 12/16 white, 3/16 yellow and 1/16 green offspring. Determine the genotypes of the parents.

3.2.8   A cross between true breeding white Leghorn and true breeding white Silkies produces all white F_1 hybrids. Numerous matings between F_1 progeny produces approximately 13/16 white and 3/16 coloured fowl. Explain the results genetically.

3.2.9   In onions, dominant gene C results in an enzyme necessary for colour production, in the presence of c, the enzyme is not produced. Another gene, I results in the inhibition of the enzyme, the allele i does not inhibit the enzyme so that colour is produced. Thus, both C and ii are necessary for colour production.

(a) What will be phenotypic ratios of the following crosses?

(i) CcIi × Ccii, (ii) Ccii × CCIi, (iii) ccII × ccii, (d) ccIi × Ccii

(b) A true breeding coloured variety of onion was crossed with a white variety having the   genotype ccII. What will be the appearance of F_1 and of the F_2 population?

3.2.10   In maize, red *aleurone* colour is dependent on two dominant genes: C and R, the absence of either results in white *aleurone*. If P is present in addition to C and R, the *aleurone* is purple, but P has no effect in the absence of either C or R or both. Find the genotype of parents and offspring in the following crosses.

(a) A purple plant crossed with a white produced offspring of which one-eighth are purple, one-eighth red and three-fourth white.

(b) A red plant crossed with a white produced offspring of which three-sixteenth are purple, three-sixteenth red and five-eighth white.

3.2.11   In swine, red coat colour is due to the presence of two dominant genes S and T, white colour is due to both recessive genes in the homozygous condition and other combination of genes result in sandy yellowish colour. What will be the genotype and phenotype in F_1 and F_2 from a cross between two sandy coat coloured mice?

3.2.12 In summer squash, two sphere-shaped varieties were crossed. The $F_1(s)$ were disc shaped. The F_2s consisted of 1/16 elongated, 3/16 sphere shaped and 9/16 disc shaped. What type of gene interaction is involved? Explain the results genetically giving reasons.

3.2.13 Red pericarp colour in wheat is dependent upon the presence of two dominant genes C_1 and C_2, colourless pericarp upon the presence of both recessive genes $c_1c_1c_2c_2$ and light red is due to presence of either C_1 or C_2. Two light red varieties were crossed. What will be the appearance of grains in F_1 and F_2 generations?

3.2.14 A cross between two yellow endosperm coloured maize varieties produced plants in the ratio of 15/16 yellow and 1/16 white endosperm. What will be the genotype of parents and offspring?

3.2.15 The F_2 progeny from a particular cross exhibit a modified dihybrids ratio of 9:7 (instead of 9:3:3:1). What phenotypic ratio would be expected from a test crossing of the F_1 individuals?

3.2.16 The inheritance of coat colour in Labrador dogs involves epistatic interaction between alleles of two loci: B (colour) and E (extension of pigment) loci as follows: Colour locus – the dominant allele 'B' causes black and its recessive allele 'b' causes brown (chocolate) coat. Extension of pigment locus – the dominant allele 'E' allows the extension of colour to hairs while its recessive allele 'e' does not permit the extension of colour to the hairs. In the absence of extension of black or brown pigment to the hairs, the coat appears yellow/golden. Thus, the homozygous recessive constitution 'ec' at the extension locus blocks the expression of both the B_ and bb genotypes causing the coat to be yellow/golden. The different genotypes responsible for the three coat-colours are:

BBEE; BBEe; BbEE; BbEe   →   B_E_ = Black

bbEE; bbEe   →   bbE_ = brown (chocolate)

BBee; Bbee; bbee   →   _ _ ee = yellow (golden)

A yellow Labrador male mated to a black Labrador bitch produced a litter containing black, brown and yellow pups. One of the brown male pups on attaining sexual maturity was mated to his dam (black), what would be the expected proportion of different coat colours among their offspring? (b) What would be the phenotypes of the offspring and in what proportions from the following matings?

(i) Brown (bbEe) × Brown (bbEe), (ii) Yellow (Bbee) × yellow (Bbee)

3.2.17 Coat colour in Duroc-Jersey breed of pigs, viz. red, sandy or white is determined by the interaction between two independently assorting loci. The red coat requires the presence of one dominant allele at each of the two loci, R and S (cumulative effect of dominant alleles of both loci). Therefore, pigs of R_S_ genotype are red. The pigs of genotypes R_ss and rrS_ (i.e., one dominant allele of either locus, but not both) are sandy. The double homozygous recessive genotype rrss produces white pigs. A mating between a red-coated male and a white-coated female, each of which came from a pure-breeding line, produces red-coated F_1. What will be the proportion of different phenotypes in the F_2 offspring produced by inter-se-mating of F_1?

3.2.18 In mice, the genes responsible for various hair colour patterns are A = pattern of banding on hair; a = recessive of A (self colour); C = colour; c = albino; E = extension of black pigment; e = restriction of black pigment to eyes. The resultant genotypes are AACCEE = pure agouti; AAccEE = albino; aaCCEE = self or solid colour; AACCee = black-eyed yellow.

(a) What types of offspring are expected from the crossing 2 and 3?

(b) What different genotypes may be obtained from those factors?

(c) Indicate eight possible genotypic kinds of agouti.

(d) What is the expectation in crossing AaCcEe and AaCcee?

(e) How many genotypically different albinos are possible from the above?

(f) How can you demonstrate that an albino is carrying the agouti pattern?

3.2.19 In mice, the genes responsible for various coat colours are U = uniformity; u = piebald (recessive of U); C = colour; and c = absence of colour (albino). The genotypes possible are UUCC = pure self-colour; UUcc = albino; uuCC = piebald; and uucc = albino.

(a) Produce the crosses: 1 × 2 = X; 1 × 3 = Y; 1 × 4 = Z

(b) Find out the result of the crosses: X × X; Y × Y; Z × Z

3.2.20 In mice, the genes and the phenotypes they cause are B = black (masking chocolate); b = chocolate; I = intensity and i = dilution. The resultant genotypes and their phenotypes are BIBI = black; BiBi = maltese (dilute black); bIbI = chocolate; bibi = silver-fawn (dilute chocolate).

(a) Cross 1 and 2 (= X). What is the phenotypic result?

(b) Cross X and X. What is the result?

(c) Cross 2 and 3. What is the result?

(d) Cross 2 and 4. What is the result?

(e) Cross 4 and 4. What is the result?

3.2.21 In poultry, the recessive (w) causes a white bird when homozygous. The genotypes WW or Ww are coloured, but only in the presence of a second gene (i). Birds of the constitution WWII or WWIi are white. When the birds of two white breeds, white Leghorns and white Plymouth Rocks are crossed, only white F_1 birds result. In the second generation, however, instead of breeding true for whites, there occurred in an actual experiment 940 coloured chicks in a flock of a total of 5000 birds.

When the F_1 birds were back-crossed to the White Plymouth Rocks, 310 whites and 99 coloured chicks resulted, but when the F_1 birds were back-crossed to the Leghorns only white progeny resulted. When coloured chicks from the first back-cross (Plymouth Rock) were bred together, there resulted 75 coloured chicks and 24 white ones. Explain, showing all the genotypes and gametes in each generation or cross. What is the genetic constitution of each of the parental breeds?

3.2.22 The white Leghorn breed of chickens is homozygous for the dominant allele C, which produces coloured feathers. However, this breed is also homozygous for the dominant allele I of an independently assorting gene that inhibits coloration of the feathers. Consequently, Leghorn chickens have white feathers. The white Wyandotte breed of chickens has neither the allele for colour nor the inhibitor of colour; it is therefore genotypically cc ii. What are the F_2 phenotypes and proportions expected from intercrossing the progeny of a white Leghorn hen and a white Wyandotte rooster?

3.2.23 Multiple crosses were made between true-breeding lines of black and yellow Labrador retrievers. All the progeny were black. When these progeny were intercrossed, they produced an F_2 consisting of 92 black, 40 yellow and 28 chocolate. Propose an explanation for the inheritance of coat colour in Labrador retrievers.

3.2.24 A lab animal breeder aimed to produce brown mice, preferably free from recessive albinism. He had five mice, black ♀; albino ♂; albino ♀; brown ♂ and black ♀. From the previous matings, he knew that 1 × 2 crosses produced albinos, blacks and browns; 3 × 4 produced all blacks and 2 × 5 had produced blacks and brown. He also knew that C = gene for either black or brown; c = albino; B = black when C is present; b = brown when C is present. Which cross will yield the greatest proportion of F_1 homozygous browns?

3.3 MULTIPLE ALLELES

Three or more genes, any one of which may occupy the same locus of homologous chromosomes in a species are called multiple alleles. All of them influence the same trait but in difference degrees; for example, coat colour in rabbits, human and animal blood groups, eye colour in Drosophila.

CLASS WORK

1. In rabbits, the wild or full colour or *agouti* (C), Himalayan (c^h) and albinism (c) form a series of multiple alleles with dominance in the order given. What will be the appearance of the offspring of the following crosses?

   (a) Full coloured × Himalayan (homozygous)
   (b) F_2 from (a)
   (c) Himalayan × albino
   (d) F_2 from (c)
   (e) F_1 from (a) × F_1 from (c)

   (a) Parents   : Full coloured   ×   Himalayan
       Genotypes   : CC $c^h c^h$
       Gametes   : C c^h
       F_1 : Cc^h
                            (All full coloured)

   (a) F_2 from (a)
       Parents   : Full coloured   ×   Full coloured
       Genotypes   : Cc^h Cc^h
       Gametes   : C c^h C c^h
       F_2 offspring : CC Cc^h Cc^h $c^h c^h$
       F_2 phenotypic ratio : 3 full coloured: 1 Himalayan

   (c) Parents   : Himalayan   ×   Albino
       Genotypes   : $c^h c^h$ cc
       Gametes   : c^h c
       Offspring   : $c^h c$
                            All Himalayan

(d) F_2 from (c)

Parents	:	Himalayan	×	Himalayan
Genotypes	:	$c^h c$		$c^h c$
Gametes	:	c^h c		c^h c
F_2 offspring	:	$c^h c^h$ $c^h c$		$c^h c$ cc

F_2 phenotypic ratio :3 Himalayan : 1 albino

(e) F_1 from (a) × F_1 from (c)

Parents	:	Full coloured	×	Himalayan
Genotypes	:	Cc^h		$c^h c$
Gametes	:	C c^h		c^h c
F_2 offspring	:	Cc^h Cc		$c^h c^h$ $c^h c$

F_2 phenotypes : 2 full coloured : 2 Himalayan

Inheritance of blood groups in human beings is an example for multiple alleles. The blood groups of parents and possible blood groups in their children are detailed in the following Table 1.

Table 1. Table showing the possible types of children among different matings

Blood groups of parents	Blood groups which may occur in children	Blood groups which do not occur in children
O × O	O	A, B, AB
O × A	O, A	B, AB
A × A	O, A	B, AB
O × B	O, B	A, AB
B × B	O, B	A, AB
A × B	O, A, B, AB	–
O × AB	A, B	O, AB
A × AB	A, B, AB	O
B × AB	A, B, AB	O
AB × AB	A, B, AB	O

HOME WORK

3.3.1   The ABO blood group system in humans exhibits multiple allelism with three major alleles, I^A, I^B and i with dominance hierarchy of $(I^A = I^B) > i$. These three alleles determine four major phenotypes or blood groups: O, A, B and AB. The results of marriages among parents of different blood groups in terms of expected genotypes and phenotypes of offspring are given below. Verify the expected genotypic and phenotypic outcome from all possible matings involving the four blood groups by making the Punnett square for each mating combination.

Blood group	Possible	
of parents	Phenotypes	Genotypes
A × A	A, O	$I^A I^A$, $I^A i$, ii
A × B	A, B, AB, O	$I^A I^B$, $I^A i$, $I^B i$, ii
A × O	A, O	$I^A i$, ii
A × AB	A, AB, B	$I^A I^A$, $I^A I^B$, $I^A i$, $I^B i$
B × B	B, O	$I^B I^B$, $I^B i$, ii
B × O	B, O	$I^B i$, ii
B × AB	B, AB, A	$I^B I^B$, $I^A I^B$, $I^A i$, $I^B i$
AB × O	A, B	$I^A i$, $I^B i$
AB × AB	A, AB, B	$I^A I^A$, $I^A I^B$, $I^B I^B$
O × O	O	ii

3.3.2   In a particular family, one parent has type A blood and the other has type B. They have four children. One has type A, one has type B, one has type AB and the last has type O. What are the genotypes of all six people in the family? (The ABO blood type gene has three alleles, I^A I^B are codominant, i is recessive to both (for type O)). A man belonging to blood type B marries a woman belonging to type A. They have four children. Their first child has blood type AB, second child has blood type O. What are the genotypes of the two individuals?

3.3.3   Assume that a trait is controlled by 'n' alleles at a locus. Give the generalized mathematical expression to calculate (a) possible number of genotypes, the number of heterozygous and homozygous genoytpes, and (b) number of possible phenotypic classes.

(Ans: (a) Possible number of genotypes for 'n' alleles = $n(n+1)/2$; possible number of heterozygotes for 'n' classes = $n(n-1)/2$ and the possible number of homozygotes for 'n' alleles = n. Check:

sum of heterozygotes and homozygotes equals $n(n+1)/2$, (b) number of phenotypic classes arising from 'n' alleles will depend upon the dominance hierarchy between the alleles. If all the alleles of the locus are codominant to each other, the number of phenotypic classes would equal the number of genotypic classes, i.e. $n(n+1)/2$. If some of the loci show complete dominance, the number of phenotypic classes will be less than the number of genotypic classes.

3.3.4   In a diploid species, a gene is known to have four alleles. (a) How many alleles would be present in: (i) one chromosome, (ii) one chromosome pair, and (iii) an individual member of the species; (b) How many different combinations of the four alleles are expected to occur in the entire population? (Ans: (a) (i) Any single chromosome can carry only one allele at a locus, (ii) a chromosome pair can carry two alleles at the corresponding place on the homologous pair, (iii) a diploid individual will carry two alleles at a locus; (b) Four alleles can give rise to 10 possible genotypic combinations (i.e., $n(n+1)/2 = (4 \times 5)/2 = 10$).

3.3.5   In mice, white-bellied agouti (A^w), agouti (A) and non-agouti (a) are alleles, A^w being dominant over both the other two. A non-agouti male is mated to two females: the first agouti and the second white-bellied agouti, and the offspring of one mating are crossed with those from the other. What results are expected?

In guinea pigs, the multiple allelic series is as follows.

C = intense colour

C_k = diluted black (chocolate) or diluted red (cream)

C_d = sepia or diluted red (yellow)

C_r = ruby-eye, destroying all other red colour

C_a = albino, destroying all colour

Order of dominance is $C > C_k > C_d > C_r > C_a$

Each animal contains two and only two of the above factors. How many different possible types of guinea pigs are there with respect to these factors, including both homozygous and heterozygous forms?

When intense-coloured guinea pigs were crossed with albinos and obtained 31 intense, 36 dilute, 0 ruby-eyed and 0 albinos, what must be the genotypes of the parents?

In an experiment, if intense-coloured guinea pigs were crossed with diluted and obtained 28 intense, 22 dilute, 0 ruby-eyed and 15 albinos, what must be the genotypes of the parents to get these results.

3.3.6   In rabbits, the alleles C, c^{ch}, c^h and c are responsible for the full colour (wild, agouti coat colour), Chinchilla, Himalayan and albino coat colours, constituting a multiple allelic series with the dominance in that order. Determine the phenotypes of the offspring of the following crosses:

(a) $Cc^h \times Cc^{ch}$	(b) $c^{ch}c \times c^hc$	(c) $Cc \times Cc$	(d) $Cc^h \times Cc$
(e) $Cc^h \times cc$	(f) $Cc^{Ch} \times Cc$	(g) $c^hc \times cc$	(h) $Cc^h \times c^hc$
(i) $CC \times cc$	(j) $Cc^h \times Cc^h$	(k) $Cc^{ch} \times cc$	

3.3.7   What blood types could be observed in children born to a woman who has blood type N and a man who has blood type M?

3.3.8   In the following cases, find out whether the child described can be actually produced from the marriage. Offer your explanation in each of the following cases.

(a) An AB child resulting from the marriage of an A to O

(b) An O child resulting from the marriage of the two individuals belonging to A group

(c) An A child from the marriage of an AB to B

(d) An O child from the marriage of an A and B

(e) An O child resulting from the marriage of an AB to A

3.3.9   A woman with type AB blood gave birth to a baby with type B blood. Two different men claim to be the father. One has type A blood, the other type O blood. Can the genetic evidence decide in favour of either?

3.3.10 A woman with type A blood gave birth to a baby, with type O blood. The woman stated that a man with type AB blood was the father of the baby. Is there any merit to her statement?

3.3.11 A woman who has blood type AB and blood type M marries a man who has blood type O and blood type MN. If we assume that the genes for the A-B-O and M-N blood-typing systems assort independently, what blood types might the children of this couple have, and in what proportions?

3.3.12 What phenotypes and ratios are expected from the following matings:

(a) I^A i × I^B I^B, (b) I^B I^B × ii, (c) I^A i × I^B I, (d) I^A i × ii

3.3.13 A man with type O blood marries a woman with type AB blood. Among their children, what proportion would you expect to have blood types like one or the other of these parents? What proportion would you expect to have blood types different from both parents? Explain.

3.3.14 In a case of disputed parentage, the results of the blood testing obtained were alleged father, type O; Mother, type A; and child, type AB. What are the possible genotypes of these three people?

3.3.15 In a hospital, it was suspected that two babies had been exchanged. In the first family, the father X (type A) and Y (type O) received baby belonging to type A; and in the second family, the father A (Type AB) and mother B (type O) and baby type O. Were the babies switched? How do you know whether they were or they were not?

3.3.16 A woman has a daughter. There are three men whom she claims might have been the father of the child. The judge in the paternity court orders that all three men, the child and the mother have blood tests. The results are as follows: mother, Type A; Daughter, Type O; Man 1, Type AB; Man 2, Type B; Man 3, Type O. The mother claims that this proves that Man 3 must be the little girl's father.

(a) Is the mother correct? Why or why not?

(b) The judge isn't satisfied, so he asks for the medical records of the people involved. He discovers that the little girl is colour blind. Men 1 and 2 are also colour blind; Man 3 has normal colour vision, as does the mother. (Colour blindness is X-linked and recessive). Assuming that one of these three men must be the father, can you now determine which of the three it is?

3.3.17 A woman's blood type is A, her child's is B. She has three candidates for fatherhood. Their blood types are Man 1 B; Man 2 AB; Man 3 O. Based on the blood types, the mother says it must have been 1. (a) Do you agree? Why or why not? (b) This child is colour blind. The only of the men in question to share this characteristic is No. 2. The mother is not colour blind. Can you now determine who the father of the little boy is, assuming it must be one of these men? Explain your answer.

3.3.18 Two independently discovered strains of mice are homozygous for a recessive mutation that causes the eyes to be small; the phenotypes of the two strains are indistinguishable. The mutation in one strain is called *little eye*, and the mutation in the other is called *tiny eye*. A third strain is heterozygous for a dominant mutation that eliminates the eyes together; the mutation in this strain is called *eyeless*. How would you determine if the *little eye*, *tiny eye* and *eyeless* mutations are alleles of the same gene?

3.4 LETHAL GENES

Lethal genes are mutant forms of normal genes. The genes which have serious effects such that they are unable to live are called lethal genes. The genes with regularly fatal effects are known as lethal genes. Lethal genes are the genes that cause death of the organism in which it occur. The death may occur either during pre-natal life or at birth. The genes which kill all or nearly all homozygous individuals before they reach sexual maturity are called *complete lethals*. The genes which kill some of the affected persons but permit others to survive long enough to have families are called *semi lethal or subvital genes*. The typical examples of lethal conditions are Achondroplacia or Bull-Dog, Amputated, short spine and hairless in cattle; paralyzed limbs, lethal muscular dystrophy, paralysis of hind limbs, lethal gray and hairlessness in sheep; paralysis of hind limbs, muscular contracture, hernia and cleft palate in swine; and sickle cell anemia, Thalassemia major, Amaurotic idiocy, epidermolysis bullosa and brachyphalangy in human beings.

CLASS WORK

1. The heterozygous Cc chickens express a condition called creeper, in which the leg and wing bones are shortened. The dominant allele C in the homozygous state CC is lethal. Skin colour is determined by independently segregating locus that exhibits complete dominance such that W are white and ww are yellow. From matings between chickens heterozygous for both the loci, what phenotypic classes will be represented among the viable progeny, and in what ratios?

    The genotypes CC are lethal, Cc are creepers, and cc are normal. Similarly, the genotypes WW and Ww results in white skin colour and ww yellow.

    Since two loci segregate independently, we can consider them as two events and then multiply. Cc × Cc will give 1 CC (lethal, die): 2 Cc : 1 cc in a ratio of 2:1 and Ww × Ww results 3 W (white) : 1 ww (yellow). Therefore, (creeper: normal: 2:1) × (white: yellow::3:1) will give 6 creeper white: 2 creeper yellow: 3 normal white: 1 normal yellow), thus 6:2:3:1. If the locus exhibiting complete dominant (skin colour) were considered first in order, the phenotypic ratio would be 3:1:6:2. Note: The problem can be solved by the branch diagram.

Segregation for creeper condition:

Parents phenotypes	:	Creeper	×	Creeper
Parents genotypes	:	Cc	×	Cc
Offspring genotypes	:	1 CC : 2 Cc : 1 cc		
Offspring phenotypes	:	1 lethal : 2 creeper : 1 normal		

Segregation for skin colour:

Parents phenotypes	:	White	×	White
Parents genotypes	:	Ww	×	Ww
Offspring genotypes	:	1 WW : 2 Ww : 1 ww		
Offspring phenotypes	:	3 white : 1 yellow		

Parents (heterozygous for both loci):

Genotypes	:	CcWw	×	CcWw
Phenotypes	:	creeper white	×	creeper white
Gametes formed	:	CW Cw cW cw × CW Cw cW cw		

Genotypes for creeper	Genotypes for skin colour	Offspring genotypes	Offspring phenotypes
CC (1/4)	WW (1/4)	CCWW (1/16)	Lethal, dies
CC (1/4)	Ww (2/4)	CCWw (2/16)	Lethal, dies
CC (1/4)	Ww (1/4)	CCww (1/16)	Lethal, dies
Cc (2/4)	WW (1/4)	CcWW (2/16)	Creeper, white
Cc (2/4)	Ww (2/4)	CcWw (4/16)	Creeper, white
Cc (2/4)	ww (1/4)	Ccww (2/16)	Creeper, yellow
cc (1/4)	WW (1/4)	ccWW (1/16)	Normal, white
cc (1/4)	Ww (2/4)	ccWw (2/16)	Normal, white
cc (1/4)	ww (1/4)	ccww (1/16)	Normal, yellow

Offspring generation: 4/16 Lethal, dies

6/16 Creeper, white : 2/16 Creeper, yellow : 3/16 Normal, white : 1/16 Normal yellow

HOME WORK

3.4.1   Determine the genotypic and phenotypic ratios resulting from each of the following dihybrid crosses (assume lethals to exert their effect during early embryo development):

Parental	Gene characteristics		Progeny ratios	
genotypes	First pair	Second pair	Genotypic	Phenotypic
(a) AaBb × AaBb	Complete dominance	Complete dominance		
(b) Aab_1b_2 × Aab_1b_2	Complete dominance	Incomplete dominance		
(c) $a_1a_2b_1b_2$ × $a_1a_2b_1b_2$	Incomplete dominance	Incomplete dominance		
(d) AaBb × AaBb	Complete dominance	Recessive lethal		
(e) a_1a_2Bb × a_1a_2Bb	Incomplete dominance	Recessive lethal		
(f) AaBb × AaBb	Recessive lethal	Recessive lethal		

Answers:

Genotypic ratios	Phenotypic ratios
(a) 1:2:1:2:4:2:1:2:1	9:3:3:1
(b) 1:2:1:2:4:2:1:2:1	3:6:3:1:2:1
(c) 1:2:1:2:4:2:1:2:1	1:2:1:2:4:2:1:2:1
(d) 1:2:1:2:4:2	3:1
(e) 1:2:1:2:4:2	1:2:1
(f) 1:2:2:4	All alike

3.4.2 The "short spine" is a lethal condition in cattle, in which the calves die shortly after birth. It is caused by homozygous recessive genotype ss. Heterozygotes are normal. A series of matings among the roan, heterozygous short-spine animals produce what phenotypic ratios at birth and after several days?

3.4.3 Work out the phenotypic ratios resulting from the cross $AaBbc_1c_2$ × $AaBbc_1c_2$ if bb is lethal and the individuals die during an early embryo stage.

3.4.4 An unnamed locus in mice is responsible for pigment production in mice. When parents heterozygous for this locus are mated together, 3/4 of the progeny are coloured and 1/4 are albino. In addition, when two yellow mice are mated together, 2/3 of the progeny are yellow and 1/3 are agouti. The albino mice cannot express whatever alleles they may have at the independently assorting agouti locus.

3.4.5   When yellow mice are crossed with albinos, they produce an F_1, consisting of 1/2 albino, 1/3 yellow and 1/6 agouti. What are the probable genotypes of the parents?

(a) If yellow F_1 mice are crossed among themselves, what phenotypic ratio would you expect among the progeny? What proportion of the yellow progeny produced would be expected to be true breeding?

3.4.6   What progeny phenotypic ratio is expected from the cross $AaBBC_1C_2 \times AaBBC_1C_2$, if bb individuals die during early embryonic stages? Assume the three loci to be assorting independently.

(Ans: Since the three loci segregate independently, consider their inheritance separately one by one and then multiply simultaneously, applying the multiplication theorem. The answer is $(3:1) \times 1 \times (1:2:1) = (3:6:3:1:2:1)$.

3.4.7   Some dogs of Mexican hairless breed are hairless, while others have normal hair. Matings between hairless and normal dogs of this breed always produce hairless and normal progeny in 1:1 ratio. In matings between two hairless dogs, hairless and normal dogs are always produced in 2:1 ratio. How can this result be explained?

(Ans: The information presented is consistent with the results that would be expected if the allele for the hairless condition is dominant, H, but lethal in the homozygous state. When this dominant allele is paired with an allele for normal hair, the recessive allele in the heterozygous state, Hh, results in hairlessness. When the dominant allele is absent altogether, as is the case, when a dog is homozygous for the normal allele, hh, normal hairs are produced.)

3.4.8   In mice, the gene for yellow (Y) is dominant over non-yellow (y). The animals homozygous for Y die in embryonic stage. The allele for naked (N) is partly dominant over normal coat (n), causing half-naked mice if heterozygous and completely naked and sterile if homozygous. What results are expected if: (a) two yellow, half-naked mice are mated; (b) a yellow, half-naked mouse is mated to a normal mouse?

3.4.9   What is the result in of a self-pollinating corn plant with the body constitution of GgRrSs when G = green foliage, g, the factor for the lack of chlorophyll (gg is lethal); R, red pericarp, r, white pericarp; S, green silks, s, salmon-coloured silks?

3.4.10   A Drosophila female homozygous for a recessive X-linked mutation which causes vermilion eyes is mated to a wild-type male with red eyes. Among their progeny, all the sons have vermilion eyes and nearly all the daughters have red eyes; however, a few daughters have vermilion eyes. Explain the origin of these vermilion-eyed daughters.

3.4.11   In fruit flies, the gene for wing shape has an unusual allele called *curly* (*Cy*). The normal wild-type allele is designated as *cy*. A fly homozygous for *cy* (*cy cy*) has normal, straight wings. The heterozygote (*Cy cy*) has the wings which curl up on the ends and cannot fly. The homozygote for the *Cy* allele (*Cy Cy*) never hatches out of the egg, as this is lethal in the homozygous condition. If two curly winged flies are mated and the female lays 100 eggs, predict the following:

(a) How many eggs will produce living offspring?

(b) How many straight winged flies do you expect among the living offspring?

(c) What percentage of the living offspring do you expect to be curly winged like the parents?

3.4.12   Thalassemia is a lethal hereditary disease in humans, which occurs in two different forms. The *thalassemia major* ($T^M T^M$) is lethal, characterized by severe anemia, enlargement of the spleen, microcytes and polycythemia. Generally such individuals die before the attainment of their sexual maturity. In *thalassemia minor* ($T^M T^N$) the erythrocytes are small (microcytic), but the affected individuals are carriers. The normal individuals are homozygous $T^N T^N$. (a) If a man with thalassemia minor ($T^M T^N$) marries a normal woman ($T^N T^N$), what proportion of their adult children is expected to be normal? (b) If both the man and woman of thalassemia minor are married, what fraction of their adult offspring would be anemic?

3.4.13 In cattle, there is an allele called *dwarf,* which, in the heterozygote, produces calves with legs which are shorter than normal. This is a homozygous lethal, and the homozygous dwarf calves spontaneously abort early or a stillborn. If a dwarf bull is mated to 400 dwarf cows, what phenotypic ratio do you expect among the living offspring?

3.4.14 In man, albinism is inherited as a simple recessive trait. Albinos lack the normal pigment of skin, hair and eyes so that their hair and skin are white and the eyes pink. Standard symbols used are C = colour, c = albino, TT = thalassemia major (severe anemia, fatal in childhood), Tt = thalassemia minor (minor anemia, often unnoticed), tt = normal blood character. The genes for thalassemia and albinism assort independently.

(a) A husband and wife, both normally pigmented and neither with severe anemia, have an albino child who dies in infancy of thalassemia major. What are the probable genotypes of the parents?

(b) If these people have another child, what are its chances of being phenotypically normal with respect to pigmentation? Of having entirely normal (non-thalessemic) blood? Of being phenotypically normal in both regards? Of being homozygous for the normal alleles of both genes?

(c) What would you expect to be the genotypic and phenotypic ratios among the children of numerous marriages?

3.4.15 The cotyledon colour in soybeans is influenced by a pair of alleles. The homozygous genotype C^GC^G produces dark green, C^GC^Y causes light green and C^YC^Y produces yellow leaves which are deficient in chloroplasts that seedlings do not grow to maturity. If dark green plants are pollinated by the light green plants and the F_1 crosses are mated to produce F_2, what phenotypic and genotypic ratios are expected in the mature F_2 soybean plants?

3.4.16 In mice, the alleles A^Y, A and a are responsible for lethal yellow, agouti (wild type) and non-agouti (black), respectively. The A^Y allele when heterozygous produces a clear yellow coat colour. However, embryos homozygous for A^Y are lethal and die and so, the F_2 phenotypic ratio will be 2 yellow: 1 black. What phenotypes and in what proportions would result from the following matings: A^Ya (yellow) × A^Y a (yellow)

$A^Y a$ (yellow) × $A^Y A$ (yellow)

$A^Y a$ (yellow) × aa (black)

$A^Y a$ (yellow) × AA (wild type)

$A^Y a$ (yellow) × Aa (wild type)

3.4.17 In Drosophila, *Dichaete* (*D*), a dominant wing-and-bristle characteristic lethal when homozygous and *Glued* (*Gl*), a dominant eye characteristic also lethal when homozygous, are so close together on the third chromosome that crossing over between the two loci is effectively absent. Given a stock of type (D Gl^+)/ (D^+ Gl), what types of progeny and in what proportions, would survive matings within the stock? Can you discern the advantages of such *"balanced lethal"* in the maintenance of *"true-breeding"* heterozygous strains?

PRACTICAL NO. 4

4.1 SEX-LINKED INHERITANCE

The genes that are located on the sex chromosomes are called sex-linked genes, and the inheritance of the traits through these genes is called as sex-linked inheritance. In addition to the autosomes, the allosomes (sex chromosomes) also carry genes for certain characters. For example, genes for eye colour in Drosophila, colour blindness and hemophilia in humans are located on the X-chromosome and show sex linkages.

Some of the sex-linked traits in poultry are rapid and slow feathering, barred and non-barred feathering, silver and gold feathering, full feathered and naked neck, and normal body and dwarf body. The heterogametic hen (ZW) transmits her sex-linked traits to her son but not to her daughter; whereas the homogametic (ZZ) cock transmits the character to both sons and daughters. This behaviour of sex-linked genes is utilized for autosexing at day-old stage. For example, when rapid feathering males (kk) are mated to hens with slow feathering (KW), all female chicks will have rapid feathering and all male chicks will be slow feathered.

One of the methods of knowing importance of sex-linked genes is to make reciprocal crosses between two strains or lines. If the sex linkage is important, the mean of two crosses approaches more towards sire line than the dam line and the reverse is true, if the maternal effects are important.

CLASS WORK

1. In Drosophila, the red eye (W) is dominant over white (w) eye and it is sex linked.
    (a) If a white-eyed female is crossed with a red-eyed male and if an F_1 female from this cross is mated with her sire and F_1 male with his dam, what would be the appearance of the offspring of these crosses?
    (b) If a white-eyed female is crossed with red-eyed male and the F_1 allowed to breed freely, what will be the appearance of F_2 with regards to the eye colour?

(a) W = red eyes; w = white eyes

Parents	:	Red-eyed male		×	White-eyed female	
Genotype	:	WY			ww	
Gametes	:	W	Y		w	w
F$_1$ offspring	:	Ww			wY	
		(all females red eyed)			(all males white eyed)	

The daughters resembling their male parent and sons resembling their female parent is known as criss-cross inheritance.

Parents	:	F$_1$ female		×	her sire	
Genotype	:	Ww			WY	
Gametes	:	W	w		W	Y
Offspring	:	WW	Ww		WY	wY
		All females		50% males	50% males	
		Red eyed		red-eyed	white-eyed	

Parents	:	F$_1$ male		×	his dam	
Genotype	:	wY			ww	
Gametes	:	w	Y		w	w
Offspring	:	ww	ww		wY	wY
		All females		All males		
		white-eyed		white-eyed		

Thus, the red-eyed male transmits the genes for red eye colour to half of his grand sons through the carrier daughters.

(b)

Parents	:	Red-eyed male		×	White-eyed female	
Genotype	:	WY			ww	
Gametes	:	W	Y		w	w
Offspring	:	Ww	Ww		wY	wY
		All females		All males		
		Red-eyed		white-eyed		

The F$_1$ flies are allowed to breed freely

Parents	:	Red-eyed female	×	White-eyed female	
Genotype	:	Ww		wY	
Gametes	:	W	w	w	Y
Offspring	:	Ww	ww	WY	wY
		50% ♀s	50% ♀s	50% ♂s	50% ♂s
		Red-eyed	white-eyed	Red-eyed	white-eyed

2. In poultry, the barred feathering (B) is dominant over non-barred feathering (b) and this character is sex linked. If a non-barred cock is crossed with a barred hen and an F_2 from this cross is allowed to interbreed freely, what will be the appearance of F_3 as to barring?

    B = barred feathering b = non-barred feathering

Parents	:	Non-barred cock	×	barred hen
Genotype	:	bb		BZ
Gametes	:	b b		B Z
F_1 offspring	:	Bb		bZ
		(Barred cock)		(Non-barred hens)
F_1 gametes	:	B b		b Z
F_2 offspring	:	Bb bb		BZ bZ
Phenotypes	:	Barred Non-barred		Barred Non-barred
		♂ ♂		♀ ♀

F_3 offspring:

Case-I

$$\text{Barred } ♂ \quad × \quad \text{Barred } ♀$$
$$\text{Bb} \qquad\qquad \text{BZ}$$

	B	b
B	BB (barred ♂)	Bb (barred ♂)
Z	BZ (barred ♀)	bZ (non-barred ♀)

Case-II

$$\text{Barred } ♂ \quad × \quad \text{Non-barred } ♀$$
$$\text{Bb} \qquad\qquad \text{bZ}$$

	B	b
b	Bb (barred ♂)	bb (non-barred ♂)
Z	BZ (barred ♀)	bZ (non-barred ♀)

Case-III

Non-barred ♂ × Barred ♀
bb   BZ

	b	b
B	Bb (barred ♂)	Bb (barred ♂)
Z	bZ (non-barred ♀)	bZ (non-barred ♀)

Case-IV

Non-barred ♂ × Non-barred ♀
bb   bZ

	b	b
b	bb (non-barred ♂)	bb (non-barred ♂)
Z	bZ (non-barred ♀)	bZ (non-barred ♀)

HOME WORK

4.1.1   A red-eyed female Drosophila was crossed to a white-eyed male. The F_1 male was back crossed to his mother and F_1 female to her father. What eye phenotype would you expect in the progeny of these crosses?

4.1.2   In man, colour blindness is due to a sex-linked recessive gene, while blue eyes are due to an autosomal recessive gene. Two brown-eyed persons with normal vision produce a blue-eyed colour blind son. What are the genotypes of the parents and offspring?

4.1.3   A woman with normal vision marries a man with normal vision. They produced a colour blind son. Give the genotypes of parents and offspring.

4.1.4   A colour blind woman marries a normal man. What kinds of children would you expect and in what proportion?

4.1.5   If a woman having normal vision has colour blind father, what is the probability that her sons will be colour blind if she marries a man with normal colour vision?

4.1.6   Barred feathering in Plymouth Rocks is due to a sex-linked dominant gene (B), while its recessive gene (b) is responsible for non-barred feathering. A non-barred hen is crossed to a barred cock. What phenotypes are expected when F_1 hen is crossed to her father cock?

4.1.7   If a father and mother have both the red-green colour blindness, is it likely that the son inherited the trait from his father?

4.1.8   In Drosophila, white eye (w) is due to a sex linked recessive gene, as against the wild red eye (W) and long wings are due to a dominant gene (V) and vestigial wings are to its recessive allele (v), but they are not sex linked.

What kinds of offspring would be expected by the following matings:

(a) wYVv × WwVv, (b) wYvv × Wwvv, (c) WYVv × WWVv, (d) WYvv × WWVV

4.1.9   In cats, the genotypes BB, Bb and bb result in black, tortoise shell and yellow coat colour, respectively. The gene is on the X-chromosome. A tortoise shell female is crossed with a black male. What offspring would be expected? Would you expect to find any tortoise shell males?

4.1.10   A normal woman, whose mother was colour blind has a son. Nothing is known of the colour-vision phenotype of the father. What is the probability that the son will be colour-blind?

4.1.11   Illustrate the following crosses among fruit flies and determine genotype and phenotypes of the resulting offspring: (a) True-breeding red-eyed female × white-eyed male (b) Heterozygous red-eyed female × white-eyed male (c) White-eyed female × red-eyed male.

4.1.12   Red- green colorblindness is caused by an X-linked recessive allele. A colorblind man marries a woman with normal vision whose father was colorblind. (a) What is the probability that their daughter will be colorblind? (b) What is the probability that they will have a colorblind son?

4.1.13   A man with hemophilia has a daughter of normal phenotype. She marries a man who is normal for the trait. (a) What is the probability that a daughter of this mating will be a hemophiliac? (b) That a son will be a hemophiliac?

4.1.14   Given that *hypophosphatemia* is an X-linked dominant trait, predict the results of the mating between: (a) An unaffected father and an affected mother (b) An affected father and an unaffected mother.

4.1.15 In mice, there is a mutant allele that causes a *bent tail*. From the cross results given in the Table below, deduce the mode of inheritance of this trait.

(a) Is it recessive or dominant?

(b) Is it autosomal or sex-linked?

(c) What are the genotypes of parents and progeny in all crosses shown in the Table?

Cross	Parents		Progeny	
	Male	Female	Male	Female
1	Bent	Normal	All normal	All bent
2	Normal	Bent	½ Bent, ½ Normal	½ Bent, ½ Normal
3	Normal	Bent	All bent	All bent
4	Normal	Normal	All normal	All normal
5	Bent	Bent	All bent	All bent
6	Bent	Bent	½ Bent, ½ Normal	All bent

4.1.16 In man, the gene (h) for hemophilia is sex-linked and recessive to the gene (h^+) for normal clotting. Diagram on the chromosomes the genotypes of the parents of the following crosses and summarize the expected phenotypic ratios resulting from the crosses: (a) hemophiliac woman × normal man; (b) normal (heterozygous) woman × hemophiliac man; (c) normal (homozygous) woman × hemophiliac man.

4.1.17 There is a dominant sex-linked gene B, which places white bars on an adult black chicken as in the Barred Plymouth Rock breed. Newly hatched chicks, which will become barred later in life, exhibit a white spot on the top of the head. (a) Diagram the cross through the F_2 between a homozygous barred male and a non-barred female. (b) Diagram the reciprocal cross through the F_2 between a homozygous non-barred male and a barred female. (c) Will both the above crosses be useful in sexing F_1 chicks at hatching?

4.1.18 In Drosophila, long wings are due to a dominant gene, V, and vestigial wings to its recessive allele, v. These are not sex-linked, whereas the white eye (w) is due to a sex-linked recessive gene, as against that of the wild red eye (W). A white-eyed, vestigial winged male is mated to homozygous red-eyed, long winged female. One of the F_1 females is crossed with the white-eyed, vestigial winged parent. What kinds of offspring will they be expected to produce and in what proportions?

4.1.19   A colour-blind woman marries a normal man. They have two children: a boy and a girl. (a) What will be the genotype and phenotype of the boy? (b) What will be the genotype and phenotype of the girl?

4.1.20   A red-eyed, long winged male Drosophila is mated to a red-eyed, vestigial winged female. They produced the following offspring:

  (a) 104 red-eyed, long-winged females

  (b) 99 red-eyed, vestigial-winged females

  (c) 101 red-eyed, long winged males

  (d) 102 red-eyed, vestigial-winged males

  What are the genotypes of the parents?

4.1.21   A normal woman, whose father was colour blind marries a normal man. What kinds of children would be expected and in what proportion?

4.1.22   A normal woman, whose father had hemophilia, marries a hemophiliac man. What is the chance that their first child will have hemophilia?

4.1.23   In Drosophila, sex of the individuals is determined by the sex index ratio, which is the ratio of number of X-chromosomes to the number of sets of autosomes. The sex index ratio of normal males is 0.5, a normal female is 1.0, super males is less than 0.5, super females is more than 1.0 and intersex between 0.5 and 1.0. What is the expected sex of Drosophila in each of the following crosses?

  (a) 3A + 2X, (b) 4A + 3X, (c) 2A + 2X, (d) 3A + 1X, (e) 2A + 3X

4.1.24   In Drosophila, an autosomal recessive gene (tra) in homozygous condition transforms normal females into sterile males. This gene has no effect in males (XY). What will be the sex ratio in a cross between a female heterozygous for tra and male homozygous recessive for same gene? What are genotypes of the parents and offspring?

4.1.25   In poultry, barring results from the dominant sex-linked gene (b^+), non-barring from its recessive allele (b). Crested head results from a dominant autosomal gene (c^+) and plain head from its recessive allele (c). Two barred, crested birds were mated and produced two offspring: a non-barred, plain female and a barred crested male. (a) Give the genotypes of the parents on the chromosomes. (b) Summarize the expected result for sex, barring and crest expressions from further matings between these two barred, crested birds.

4.1.26 In Drosophila, white eyes is a sex-linked character. The mutant allele for white eyes (w) is recessive to the wild-type allele for brick red eye colour (w^+).

(a) A white-eyed female is crossed with a red-eyed male, and an F_1 female from this cross is mated with her father and an F_1 male is mated with her mother. What will be the appearance of the offspring of these last two crosses with respect to the eye colour?

(b) A white-eyed female is crossed with a red-eyed male, and the F_1 from this cross is interbred. What will be appearance of the F_3 with respect to eye colour?

4.1.27 A man with a hereditary vision defect marries a phenotypically normal woman. They have eight children, four boys with normal vision and four girls with the same vision defect as their father. What does this suggest about the genetic basis of the trait, with respect to whether it is dominant or recessive and autosomal, X-linked or Y-linked?

4.1.28 The *vermilion* eye colour of Drosophila is determined by the recessive allele v of an X-linked gene; the wild-type eye colour produced by the v^+ allele is brick red. What phenotypic ratios are expected from the crosses: (a) vermilion female × wild-type male, (b) homozygous wild-type female × vermilion male and (c) heterozygous female × vermilion male?

4.1.29 The male house cats are either black or yellow; females are black, tortoise-shell pattern or yellow.

(a) If these colours are governed by a sex-linked gene, how can these observations be explained?

(b) Using appropriate symbols, determine the phenotypes expected in the progeny of a cross between a yellow female and a black male.

(c) Repeat part b for the reciprocal of the cross described there.

(d) One-half of the females produced by certain kind of mating are tortoise-shell and one-half are black; one-half of the males are yellow and one-half are black. What colours are the parental males and females in this kind of mating?

(e) Another kind of mating produces progeny in the following proportions: ¼ yellow males, ¼ yellow females, ¼ black males and ¼ tortoise-shell females. What colours are the parental males and females in this kind of mating? A female fowl which has become converted into a male producing sperm and developed male secondary sex characters, if such a male is mated to a normal female, what sex ratio would be expected in the progeny?

4.1.30   What is the sex phenotype of the following human genotypes:

(a) XXY   (b) XXYY   (c) XXXY   (d) XO   (e) XXX

4.1.31   Yellow body colour in Drosophila is controlled by a sex-linked recessive gene, y. The dominant allele Y produces wild-type body colour. State the phenotypic ratios from the following crosses:

(a) Yellow ♀ × wild type ♂

(b) Yellow ♀ × yellow ♂

(c) Wild-type ♀ (homozygous) × yellow ♂

(d) Daughter from mating of Wild-type ♀ (homozygous) × yellow ♂ with wild type ♂

(e) Daughter from mating of Wild-type ♀ (homozygous) × yellow ♂ with yellow ♂

4.1.32   Red-green colour blindness in humans is caused by a sex-linked recessive gene, r. A colour-blind man marries a normal vision woman whose father was colour-blind. (a) What is the possible genotype of the normal-vision woman? (b) What is the possible genotype of the mother of the colour-blind man? (c) Determine the phenotypic ratios in the offspring of this marriage (both sexes). (d) What fraction of all the girls produced are expected to be (i) colour-blind? (ii) carrier of colour-blindness?

Prove that all the sons of a colour-blind mother will be colour-blind irrespective of the father's vision.

4.1.33   The black and yellow pigments in the fur of cats are determined by an X-linked pair of co-dominant alleles: c^b (black) and c^y (yellow). Males can be black (c^bY) or yellow (c^yY), the homozygous c^bc^b;

females are black, the homozygous $c^y c^y$; females are yellow and heterozygous $c^b c^y$; females exhibit patches of black and yellow, a pattern known as *calico*.

(a) What genotypes and phenotypes would be expected among the offspring of a cross between a black female and a yellow male?

(b) In a litter of seven kittens, there are two calico females, one yellow female, two black males, and two yellow males. What are the genotypes and phenotypes of the parents?

(c) Calico males that result from the non-disjunction of sex chromosomes are also rarely obtained. What can be their sex-chromosome constitution and the genotype?

4.1.34 Hemophilia in dogs is controlled by a sex-linked recessive allele, h. A dog fancier has a normal-clotting prized bitch that came from hemophilic father. The fancier intends to mate her to a normal blood-clotting male and plans to have a large number of pups over a series of matings. Should he expect to have any hemophilic pups? If so, give the sex of those affected and their expected frequency. (Ans: Male; ¼ of all offspring)

4.1.35 Red-green colour-blindness in humans is due to a sex-linked recessive allele. A couple, normal for colour vision, had a colour-blind son. What are the genotypes of husband and wife? (Ans: Man is RY, woman is Rr.)

4.1.36 A prized Labrador dog having an abnormality of skin is mated with a normal bitch. They produced 16 pups (8 males and 8 females) over two crops. All of the daughters had their father's disease but none of the sons had the skin disease. Which of the following type of inheritance is suggested? (Ans: X-linked dominant)

(a) Autosomal recessive, (b) autosomal dominant, (c) Y-linked, (d) X-linked dominant, (e) X-linked recessive

4.1.37 A man is heterozygous (Bb) for an autosomal locus and is carrier of a recessive X-linked allele, d. What proportion of his sperm will be carrying the 'bd' combination? (Ans: ¼)

4.1.38 In grasshoppers, rosy body colour is caused by a recessive mutation; the wild-type body colour is green. If the gene for body colour is on the X-chromosome, what kind of progeny would be obtained from a mating between a homozygous rosy female and a hemizygous wild-type male? (In grasshoppers, females are XX and males are XO).

4.1.39 In humans, the recessive X-linked mutation, g, causes green-defective colour vision; the wild-type allele G causes normal colour vision. A man (a) and a woman (b), both with normal vision, have three children, all married to people with normal vision: a colour-defective son (c), who has a daughter with normal vision (f); a daughter with normal vision (d), who has one colour-defective son (g) and two normals (h); and a daughter with normal vision (e), who has six normal sons (i). Give the most likely genotypes for the individuals (a to i) in this family.

4.1.40 In the mosquito *Anopheles culifaciens*, *golden* body (*go*) is a recessive X-linked mutation and *brown* eyes (*bw*) is a recessive autosomal mutation. A homozygous XX female with brown eyes mated to a hemizygous XY male with golden body. Predict the phenotypes of their F_1 offspring. If the F_1 progeny are intercrossed, what kinds of progeny will appear in the F_2 and in what proportions?

4.1.41 The Drosophila females that had white eyes and ebony bodies were crossed to wild-type males, which had red eyes and gray bodies. Among the F_1, all the daughters had red eyes and gray bodies and all the sons had white eyes and gray bodies. These flies were intercrossed to produce F_2 progeny, which were classified for eye and body colour and then counted. Among 384 total progeny, the geneticist obtained the following results:

Phenotypes

Eye colour	Body colour	Males	Females
White	Ebony	20	21
White	Gray	70	73
Red	Ebony	28	25
Red	Gray	76	71

How would you explain the inheritance of eye colour and body colour?

(Ans: The results in the F_1 tell us that both mutant phenotypes are caused by recessive alleles. Furthermore, because the males and females have different eye colour phenotypes we know that the eye colour gene is X-linked and that the body colour gene is autosomal. In the F_2, the two genes assort independently, as we would expect for genes located on different chromosomes. In the following Table, the genotypes of the different classes of flies in this experiment using w for the white mutation and e for the ebony mutation the wild-type alleles are denoted by plus signs. Following the convention of Drosophila geneticists, the sex chromosomes are written on the left and the autosomes on the right. A question mark in the genotype indicates that either the wild-type or mutant alleles could be present.

Phenotypes		Genotypes	
Eye colour	Body colour	Males	Females
White	Ebony	w/Y e/e	w/w e/e
White	Gray	w/Y +/?	w/w +/?
Red	Ebony	+/Y e/e	+/w e/e
red	Gray	+/Y +/?	+/w +/?

4.1.42 In Drosophila, the gene for bobbed bristles (recessive allele, bb, bobbed bristles, wild-type allele+, normal bristles) is located on the X-chromosome and on a homologous segment of the Y-chromosome. Give the genotypes and phenotypes of the offspring from the following crosses:

(a) $X^{++} X^{++} \times X^{bb} Y^+$ (b) $X^{bb} X^{bb} \times X^{bb} Y^+$ (c) $X^+ X^{bb} \times X^+ Y^{bb}$ (d) $X^+ X^{bb} \times X^{bb} Y^+$

4.1.43 In Drosophila, vermilion eye colour (v) is due to a recessive allele located on the X-chromosome. Curved-wings is due to a recessive allele (cu) located on an autosome, and *ebony* body is due to a recessive allele (e) located on another autosome. A vermilion male is mated to a curved, ebony female, and the F_1 males are phenotypically wild type. If these males are backcrossed to curved, *ebony* females, what proportion of the F_2 offspring will be wild-type males?

4.1.44 A Drosophila female, heterozygous for the recessive X-linked mutation w (for *white eyes*) and its wild-type allele w+ is mated to a male with white eyes. Among the sons, half have white eyes and half have red eyes. Among the daughters, some have red eyes; and some have white eyes. Explain the origin of these white-eyed daughters.

4.1.45 A man with X-linked colour blindness marries a woman with no history of colour blindness in her family. The daughter of this couple marries a normal man, and their daughter also marries a normal man. What is the chance that this last couple will have a child with colour blindness? If this couple has already had a child with colour blindness, what is the chance that their next child will be colour blind?

4.1.46 A man who has colour blindness and type A-blood has children with a woman who has normal colour vision and type O-blood. The woman's father had colour blindness. Colour blindness is determined by an X-linked gene and blood type is determined by an autosomal gene.

(a) What are the genotypes of the man and the woman?

(b) What proportion of their children will have colour blindness and type B-blood?

(c) What proportion of their children will have colour blindness and type A-blood?

(d) What proportion of their children will be colour blind and have type AB blood?

4.1.47 In chickens, absence of barred feathers is due to a recessive allele. A barred rooster was mated with a non-barred hen and all the offspring were barred. These F_1 chickens were intercrossed to produce F_2 progeny, among which all the males were barred, half the females were barred and half were non-barred. Are these results consistent with the hypothesis that the gene for barred feathers is located on one of the sex chromosomes?

4.1.48 A Drosophila male carrying a recessive X-linked mutation for yellow body was mated to a homozygous wild-type female with gray body. The daughters of this mating all have uniformly gray bodies. Why are not their bodies a mosaic of yellow and gray patches?

4.1.49 In fruit flies (Drosophila), the eye colour gene is X-linked, with a recessive white allele (w) and a dominant red allele (W). If white-eyed female flies are bred to red-eyed male flies, describe the expected offspring (assume all parental flies are true breeding). What results do you expect if you do the reciprocal cross (reverse the phenotypes of the parent flies)?

4.1.50 A man with normal eye vision marries a colour blind woman. The normal allele is dominant to the colour blindness allele. If they have a large family, in what ways should the colour blindness trait affect their children?

4.1.51 A colour blind man marries a woman who is homozygous for the normal colour vision allele. If they have eight children, how many of them would you expect to be colour blind? Using Punnett's squares, derive and compare the genotypic and phenotypic ratios expected for the offspring of this marriage.

4.1.52 A normal vision woman had colour blind father and colour blind maternal grandfather (her mother's father). This woman marries a colour blind man and they just had their first child, a son. Answer the following questions about this small family.

(a) What is the probability that this child will be colour blind?

(b) Three sources of colour blindness allele are mentioned in this family. If the child just born is colour blind, from which of these three men (woman's grandfather, woman's father and father) did he inherit the allele?

(c) Using proper pedigree format, diagram the available information about the four generations of this family described, assuming that the child is colour blind.

(d) If the child's father was not colour blind, how would this affect the prediction about the newborn child?

4.1.53 In cats, there is a coat colour gene, which is located on the X-chromosome, has two alleles: orange and black. A heterozygous cat of these two alleles has tortoiseshell colour (a splotchy mixture of orange and black). Predict the genotypic and phenotypic frequencies among the offspring of the following crosses:

(a) Black female × Orange male

(b) Orange female × Black male

(c) Tortoiseshell female × Black male

(d) Tortoiseshell female × Orange male

4.1.54 Red-Green colour blindness is a sex-linked recessive trait. A woman with normal vision, whose father was colour blind marries a man with normal vision. What is the genotype of each of these people?

4.1.55 Hemophilia is a disease caused by a recessive trait on the X-chromosome. Assume you are a Genetic Counselor. Bob and his sister Mary come to your office. Bob is 25 years and has no children. Mary is 23 and engaged. However, they had a brother and uncle who died of hemophilia. Bob and Mary both want to know what are their chances of having hemophiliac children. What would you say to them?

4.1.56 In man, hemophilia (*bleeder's disease*) is due to a sex-linked recessive gene, in which the time required for the blood to clot is greatly prolonged. In the following questions, let h^+ = the allele for normal clotting time; h = the allele for hemophilia.

(a) A man, whose father was hemophilic, but whose own blood clotting time is normal, marries a normal woman with no record of hemophilia in her ancestry. What is the chance of hemophilia in their children?

(b) A woman, whose father was hemophilic, but who is not herself a *bleeder*, marries a normal man. What is the chance of hemophilia in their children?

4.1.57 A certain form of muscular dystrophy is inherited as a sex-linked recessive gene. Jack has muscular dystrophy (Neither of his parents has this disease). Jane, Jack's wife, does not have muscular dystrophy, but her father does. What fraction of their granddaughters would you expect to have muscular dystrophy? What fraction of their sons would you expect to have muscular dystrophy?

4.1.58 Colour blindness is due to a sex-linked recessive gene. A colour blind woman marries a man with normal vision. She is pregnant. What is the chance that her child will be: (a) a girl with normal vision? (b) A colour blind girl? (c) A boy with normal vision? (d) A colour blind boy?

(a) Why are men never heterozygous for an X-linked trait?

(b) Why must men always inherit an X-linked trait from their mothers?

(c) Can a colour blind father pass this allele on to his son? Explain.

(d) Can a normal male ever have a daughter that is colour blind? Explain.

4.1.59 Anthony, a colour blind person, got married, divorced and remarried. He and his first wife, Linda, have a colour blind son, a colour blind daughter, a normal son and a normal daughter. He and his current wife, Mary, have four boys and two girls, none of whom is colour blind. Give the genotype of each wife and state whether or not she is colour blind.

4.1.60 A recessive mutation in an X-linked gene causes hemophilia, characterized by a prolonged increase in blood clotting time. Suppose that two phenotypically normal parents produce three normal daughters and a son affected with hemophilia, (a) what is the probability that all the daughters are heterozygous carriers, and (b) if one of the daughters marries a normal male and produces a son, what is the probability that the son is hemophilic?

(Answer: (a) Since the phenotypically normal parents have an affected son who gets his only X chromosome from his mother, mother must be a carrier of the mutation. Therefore, the probability that any daughter is a carrier is ½. The probability that all the three daughters are carriers is $(½)^3$ because their births are independent.

If the daughter is not a carrier, the probability of an affected son is zero; and if the daughter is a carrier, the probability of an affected son is ½. Because the probability of the daughter being a carrier is ½, the overall probability of getting a son is (½) × 0 + (½) × (½) = ¼.)

4.1.61 A woman who is heterozygous for two mutations of phenylketonuria and hemophilia has married a phenotypically normal man who is also heterozygous for phenylketonuria mutation. They have a child. What is the probability that the child will be affected by both the diseases with an assumption that the parents are equally likely to have a son or daughter?

4.1.62 A normal woman (chromosomally) and normal man (chromosomally) have a son, whose sex chromosome constitution is XXY. In which parent and in which meiotic division did the non-disjunction take place?

4.1.63 The tall, yellow-flowered plants were mated with short, white-flowered plants. Both varieties are true breeding. The resultant F_1 plants were backcrossed to white, short-flowered ones. This backcross has produced 800 progeny in the proportions of 234 tall, yellow; 203 tall, white; 175 short, yellow; and 188 short, white plants. Test whether the observed ratio fit the hypothesis of 1:1:1:1 segregation ratio.

4.2 SEX-INFLUENCED INHERITANCE

The genes for sex-influenced inheritance are carried on the autosomes, and their expression is influenced by the sex of the individual. In the heterozygotes, the genes usually are expressed as dominant in the male and as recessive in the female. The inheritance of coat colour in Ayrshire cattle, horns in sheep and baldness in human beings are good examples of the sex-influenced traits. The following Table gives the genotypes and phenotypes for these traits.

Trait/genotype	Phenotype of the males	Phenotype of the females
Coat colour in Ayrshire cattle:		
MM	Mahogany and white	Mahogany and white
Mm	Mahogany and white	Red and white
mm	Red and white	Red and white
Horns in sheep:		
HH	Horned	Horned
Hh	Horned	Hornless
Hh	Hornless	Hornless
Baldness in human beings:		
BB	Bald	Bald
Bb	Bald	Non-bald
bb	Non-bald	Non-bald

CLASS WORK

1. Baldness (B) in man is dominant to normal hair but recessive in woman. A non-bald woman, whose mother was bald, marries a bald-headed man. What may be expected in their children?

   B = bald, b = normal hair (non-bald)

   Possible genotypes of bald-man are BB or Bb

   Possible genotypes of non-bald woman are Bb or bb

Non-bald woman	×	Bald man
(Bb or bb)		(BB or Bb)

Mother of this woman was bald.

Possible genotype is only BB. Hence, one B gene from this bald woman will be passed on to her daughter. Therefore, the genotype of woman must be Bb.

$$Bb \quad \times \quad \text{either BB or Bb}$$

The possible children are:

Bb × BB gives 1/2 BB : 1/2 Bb. Both bald and non-bald children are expected in a ratio of 50:50.

Bb × Bb gives 1/4 BB: 1/2 Bb: 1/4 bb, again bald and non-bald children.

HOME WORK

4.2.1   A couple has four children. Neither the father nor the mother is bald; one of the two sons is bald, but neither of the daughters is bald. (a) If one of the daughters marries a bald man and they have a son, what is the chance that the son will become bald as an adult? (b) If the couple has a daughter, what is the chance that she will not be bald as an adult?

4.2.2   The pattern of baldness in humans depends on an allele recessive to its normal alternative in women but dominant in men. Thus, the genotype B_1B_1 is non-bald in men and women, B_2B_2 is bald in both men and women, while the genotype B_1B_2 expressed as bald in men and non-bald in women.

(a) A bald woman marries a non-bald man. What is the probability that a son of theirs will be bald? A daughter?

(b) A non-bald woman whose mother was bald marries a bald man whose father was non-bald. What is the probability that a son of theirs will be bald? A daughter?

(c) A non-bald woman whose mother was bald marries a non-bald man. What is the probability that a son of theirs will be bald? A daughter?

4.2.3   In some breeds of sheep, both the males and females have horns; while in some other breeds, both sexes are hornless. When some of these breeds are crossed, the F_1 males are all horned while the F_1 females are all hornless. Suggest a simple hypothesis which would explain this situation.

4.2.4   Find out the appearance of F_2 individuals if the F_1(s) are produced in the above pattern.

(a) What genotypes and phenotypes are expected if F_1 rams are back crossed to ewes of the hornless parent breed? If this ram is crossed back to ewes of horned parent breed?

(b) What genotypes and phenotypes are expected if the F_1 ewes are crossed back with a ram of the horned parent breed? If F_1 ewes are bred to the rams of the hornless parent breed?

4.2.5   Spotting in cattle is controlled by two alleles where CM is the allele for mahogany and white, while CR is the allele for red and white. This trait is sex-influenced and the different sexes exhibit the two phenotypes as follows:

In males:

(a) Mahogany and white a dominant (CMCM, CMCR)

(b) Red and white a recessive (CRCR)

In females:

(a) Red and white a dominant (CRCR, CMCR)

(b) Mahogany and white (CMCM)

(1) If a red and white male is crossed to a mahogany and white female, what phenotypic and genotypic proportions are expected in the F_1 and F_2 generations?

(2) If a mahogany and white cow gives birth to a red and white calf, what sex is the calf?

4.2.6   In sheep, the gene H behaves as dominant and produces horns in male and recessive in females with no horns. A hornless female was crossed to a horned male. What is the chance that F_2 males and females will produce horns?

4.3 SEX-LIMITED INHERITANCE

Some hereditary traits in farm animals are limited to only one sex and therefore, they are called sex-limited traits. For example, bulls do not produce milk and cocks do not lay eggs but the males do possess and transmit the genes for these traits to their offspring. Practically, when a polygenic trait is limited to only one sex, it becomes difficult to locate the males carrying superior genes for such trait. The records of close relative of the male help to determine his genetic potential for a trait. Such females include his mother, sisters and daughters.

CLASS WORK

In poultry, the appearance of certain feather patterns is limited to males, who can be either cock-feathered or hen-feathered, depending on their genotypes. Females, on the other hand, are hen-feathered no matter what their genotype is. If 'F' represents the dominant gene and 'f' represents the recessive gene for this character, furnish the genotype for each of the following pairs of parents:

(a)	Parents	Hen-feathered male × hen-feathered female
	Offspring	Males: ¾ hen-feathered; ¼ cock-feathered
		Females: all hen-feathered
(b)	Parents	Cock-feathered male × hen-feathered female
	Offspring	Males: all cock feathered
		Females: all hen-feathered
(c)	Parents	Hen-feathered male × hen-feathered female
	Offspring	Males: ½ cock-feathered; ½ hen-feathered
		Females: all hen-feathered
(d)	Parents	Cock-feathered male × hen-feathered female
	Offspring	Males: ½ cock-feathered; ½ hen-feathered
		Females: all hen-feathered

(a) F = cock feathered; f = hen-feathered

Hen-feathered female may be either FF or Ff while the cock-feathered male must have the genotype ff only.

$$F\_ \quad \times \quad F\_ \text{ or ff}$$

$$\downarrow$$

In case of ♂ progeny : 3/4th hen-feathered

1/4th cock-feathered

In case of ♀ progeny : all hen-feathered

Among the male progeny, one-fourths are cock-feathered. Therefore, both parents must carry one f gene. Hence, the genotype of male parent is Ff and that of the females' will be ff.

(b) The genotype of hen-feathered male is ff. Since all the male offspring are cock-feathered, the female parent must carry the dominant F gene. Therefore, the genotype of female can be FF or Ff.

(c) Class work

(d) Class work

HOME WORK

4.3.1   In domestic fowl, the differences in plumage between males and females are sex influenced. If the genotypes and phenotypes for plumage are as listed below:

Genotype	Phenotype in males	Phenotype in females
HH	Hen feathered	Hen feathered
Hh	Hen feathered	Hen feathered
hh	Rooster (cock) feathered	Hen feathered

Predict the F_1 and F_2 results of crossing a male that is rooster feathered and a true-breeding hen-feathered female.

4.3.2   In the clover butterfly, all males are yellow, but females may be yellow if they are of the homozygous recessive phenotype (yy), or white if they possess the dominant allele (Y_). What phenotypic proportions are expected from a cross between heterozygous parents?

4.4 SEX DETERMINATION

Sex of the individuals in humans is determined by the number of X-chromosomes or by the presence or absence of Y-chromosome. The maleness is due to a dominant effect of the Y chromosome, which is evident by the fact that the individuals with XO develop as females and XXY individuals develop as males. The dominant effect of Y-chromosome is manifested early in development, when it directs the primordial gonads to develop into testes. The sexual identity of an individual is determined at several levels, chromosomal sex, gonadal sex, somatic sex and sexual orientation.

In human beings sex is determined by the X- and Y-chromosomes. A female is XX (homogametic) and male is XY (heterogametic). In Drosophila, the ratio of X-chromosomes to the autosomes (X/A) determines the sex of the individual flies. X-chromosomes favour femaleness, while the autosomes favour maleness. In *Malandrium*, Y-chromosome is important for male flowers. In honeybees and wasps, sex is determined by haploid and diploid chromosome numbers. In *Bonellia*, a marine worm, sex is modified due to environment in which larva develops. A single gene is responsible for sex determination in maize.

The testis-determining factor (TDF) is the product of a gene called SRY (for sex-determining region Y), which is located just outside the pseudoautosomal region in the short arm of the Y-chromosome. The discovery of SRY was made possible by the identification of unusual individuals whose sex was inconsistent with their chromosome constitution: XX males and XY females. Some of the XX males were found to carry a small piece of the Y-chromosome inserted into one of the X-chromosomes. This piece carried a gene responsible for maleness. Similarly, some of the XY females were found to carry an incomplete Y-chromosome. The part of the Y chromosome that was missing corresponded to the piece that was present in XX males; its absence in the XY females apparently prevented them from developing testes. These complementary lines of evidence showed that a particular segment of the Y-chromosome was needed for male development.

Sex determination and chromosomes

Organism	XX	XY	Other
Human	Female	Male	
Birds	Male	Female	
Grasshopper	Female		Male X-, (no Y-chromosome)
Bee			Diploid female; Haploid male
Drosophila			Sex-index ratio, balance ratio between the sets of X-chromosomes and autosomes

HOME WORK

4.4.1   A woman carries the testicular feminization mutation (*tfm*) on one of her X-chromosomes; the other X-chromosome carries the wild-type allele (*Tfm*). If this woman marries a normal man, what fraction of her children will be phenotypically female? Of these, what fraction will be fertile?

4.4.2   Predict the sex of Drosophila with the following chromosome compositions (A=number of haploid sets of autosomes):

(a) 4X 4A (b) 3X 4A (c) 4X 5A (d) 1X 3A (e) 6X 6A (f) 1X 2A

4.4.3   What are the sexual phenotypes of the following genotypes in Drosophila: XX, XY, XXY, XXX, XO?

4.4.4   Find out the maximum number of Barr bodies in the nuclei of human cells with the following sex chromosome compositions.

(a) XY (b) XX (c) XXY (d) XXXX (e) XXXXX (f) XXYY

4.4.5   Identify the sexual phenotypes of the following genotypes in human beings: XX, XY, XO, XXX, XXY, XYY.

PRACTICAL NO. 5

5.1 LINKAGE AND CHROMOSOME MAPPING

When two or more genes are on the same chromosome, they are said to be linked. Genes on different chromosomes are distributed into gametes independently of one another (Mendel's law of independent assortment). Genes on the same chromosome, however, tend to stay together during the formation of gametes. Thus, the results of test crossing dihybrid individuals will yield different results.

Example

Genes on different chromosomes assort independently, giving a 1:1:1:1 test cross ratio.

Parents   :   AaBb   ×   aabb

Gametes   :   AB   Ab   aB   ab   ab

F_1 :   ¼ AaBb   :   ¼ Aabb   :   ¼ aaBb   :   ¼ aabb

The linked genes do not assort independently but tend to stay together in the same combinations as they were in the parents. Genes to the left of the slash line (/) are on one chromosome and those to the right are on the homologous chromosomes.

Parents   :   AB/ab   ×   ab/ab

Gametes   :   AB   ab   ab

F_1 :   ½ AB/ab   :   ½ ab/ab

The deviations from a 1:1:1:1 ratio in the test cross progeny of a dihybrid could be used as an evidence for linkage. Linked genes do not always stay together, because homologous non-sister chromatids may exchange segments of varying length with one another during meiotic prophase. The homologous chromosomes pair with one another during synapsis, form chiasmata and produce recombinant gametes through crossing over.

Crossing Over

During Meiosis, each chromosome replicates, forming two identical sister chromatids. The homologous chromosomes pair and crossing over occurs between non-sister chromatids. This process involves the breakage and reunion of only two of the four strands at any given point on the chromosomes.

Coupling and Repulsion Phase

The alleles of double heterozygotes (dihybrids) at two linked loci may appear in either of two positions relative to each other. If the two dominant (or wild type) alleles are on one chromosome and the two recessive (or mutant) on the other (AB/ab), the linkage relationship is called *coupling phase*. When the dominant allele of one locus and the recessive allele of other occupy the same chromosome (Ab/aB), the relationship is termed *repulsion phase*.

Chiasma Frequency

The longer the chromosome, the greater is the number of chiasmata. Each type of chromosome within a species has a characteristic number of chiasmata. The farther apart two genes are located on a chromosome, the greater the opportunity for a chiasma to occur between them. The closer the two genes are located, the smaller the chance for a chiasma occurring between them. The chiasma frequency is useful in predicting the proportions of parental and recombinant gametes expected to be formed from a given genotype. The percent crossover gametes formed by a given genotype is the reflection of the frequency with which chiasma forms between the genes in question. The crossing over is detected only when a crossover forms between the genes under consideration.

When a chiasmata form between two genes, only half of the gametes formed will be of crossover type. Therefore, chiasma frequency is twice the frequency of crossover products.

Chiasma % = 2 (crossover %) or Crossover % = ½ (chiasma %)

Example: If a chiasma forms between the genes A and B in 30% of the gametes in an individual of the genotype AB/ab, then 15% of the gamete will be recombinant (Ab or aB) and 85% will be parental (AB/ab).

Limits of Recombination

If two loci are located such a far apart on a chromosome that the probability of a chiasma forming between them is 100 percent, then 50% of the gametes will be of parental (non-crossover) type. When such dihybrid individuals are crossed, they are expected to produce the progeny in 1:1:1:1 ratio as would be expected for genes on different chromosomes. Recombination between two linked genes cannot exceed 50% even when multiple crossovers occur between them.

The expected frequency of DCO should be the product of the frequency of the two single crossovers since the probability of simultaneous occurrence of two independent events is the product of their separate probabilities. For example, if the frequency of single crossover between y and ec was 0.054 and between ec and ct was 0.203, then the expected frequency of DCO is $0.054 \times 0.203 = 0.011$ or 1.10 per cent. The observed frequency of DCO was 0.34 percent. Hence, the coincidence, the ratio between observed DCO to expected DCO, is $0.34 \div 1.10 = 0.31$, i.e. only 31 percent of the expected double crossovers were found with an interference of 69 percent.

Genetic Mapping

The linkage of genes in a chromosome can be represented in the form of a genetic map, which shows the linear order of the genes along the chromosome with the distances between adjacent genes proportional to the frequency of recombination between them. A genetic map is also called as a linkage map or chromosome map. The concept of genetic mapping was first developed by Morgan's student Alfred H. Sturtevant in 1913.

(1) Map distance

The distance between genes in a genetic map is measured in map units. One map unit equals one percent recombination. For example, two genes recombine with a frequency of 3.5 percent are said to be located 3.5 map units apart. One map unit is also called centimorgan (abbreviated cM), in honor of T.H. Morgan. A distance of 3.5 map units therefore equals 3.5 centimorgans and indicates 3.5 percent recombination between the genes. For easy understanding, the four ways in which genetic distance between two genes may be represented are as follows: frequency of recombination (for example 0.035); percent recombination (3.5 percent); map distance in map units (3.5 map units); and map distance in centimorgans (3.5 centimorgans, abbreviated cM). Physically, one map unit can be defined as the length of the chromosome in which on an average, one crossover is formed in every 50 cells undergoing Meiosis.

The places where genes located on the chromosome (loci) are positioned in linear order like beads on a string. The two major aspects of genetic mapping are (i) determination of the linear order of the genes (gene order) and (ii) determination of the relative distances between the genes (gene distances). The unit of distance is an expression of the probability that crossover will occur between the two genes under consideration.

(2) Two-point test cross

Suppose, we test cross dihybrid individuals in coupling phase (AC/ ac) and find in the progeny phenotypes 37% dominant at both loci (AC/

ac), 37% recessive at both loci (ac/ac), 13% dominant at first locus and recessive at second locus (Ac/ac) and 13% dominant at second locus and recessive at first locus (aC/ac). The last two groups (Ac/ac and aC/ac) are produced by crossover gametes from the dihybrid parent. Thus, 26% of all the gametes produced were crossover type and the distance between the loci a and c is estimated to be 26 map units.

(3) Three-point test cross

Bridges and Olbrycht developed a technique called 'three point test cross' in *Drosophila melanogaster* by taking three genes at a time which were all linked, i.e. present on the same chromosome and crossed to their mutant recessive parents. The F_1 hybrid obtained was heterozygous for the wild (+) and mutant genes. This F_1 hybrid was test crossed with the triple-recessive parent and obtained eight different test cross progeny, since it was trihybrid. The experiment is as follows:

The mutant recessive genes and their phenotypes are ec-echinus (rough eyes), sc-scute (certain bristles missing on the body) and cv-crossveinless (absence of cross veins in the wings). In contrast, the wild-type genes are Ec – non-rough eyes; Sc – all bristles present and CV – cross veins present. All the genes are sex linked. The hybrid F_1 females are all normal, and on one X-chromosome the genes sc, cv, + are present and on the other X-chromosome, the genes ec, + + are carried. Thus, the genotype of F_1 females is (+ ec +/ sc + cv). These F_1 females are test crossed to the males with three recessive genes: sc, ec, cv, and produce 8 test cross progeny in equal proportions. But the parental combinations were more predominant than the crossover combinations. The phenotypes, genotypes and the number of flies produced are:

Phenotype	Genotype	No. of flies	Total	Remarks
Echinus	+ ec +	810		
Scute, crossveinless	sc + cv	828	1638	Parental combinations
Scute, echinus	sc ec +	62		
Crossveinless	+ + cv	88	150	Crossovers
Scute	sc + +	89		
Echinus, crossveinless	+ ec cv	103	192	Crossovers
Wild type	+ + +	0		
Scute, echinus, crossveinless	sc ec cv	0	0	Double crossovers

The first step in computing the map distances on the chromosome is to identify the parental combinations, which can be done by looking at the largest numbers among the test cross progeny. The echinus (810), scute and crossveinless (828) are the parental combinations. Then the lowest number has to be looked into. Here, the wild type (+ + +) and scute, echinus, crossveinless (*sc* ec cv) is zero. These are the double crossovers (DCOs).

The second step is to find the gene sequence. This can be done by taking the parental combinations and by drawing the two chromosomes with the given sequence in the problem. If the expected DCOs obtained by putting the double crossover between region I and region II are the same as the double crossovers given in the question, then it can be confirmed that the given gene sequence, i.e. *sc* ec cv, is correct. If not obtained, rearrange the genus on the parental combinations.

The third step is to identify the crossovers in the region I by marking one crossover between the region I. In the given problem, the scute, echinus and crossveinless are the crossovers at region I. In the next step identify the crossovers in the region II. Like this, all the eight test cross progenies are identified into the parental combinations, crossovers at the regions I and II and the double crossovers.

The percent crossovers at region I (between *sc*-ec) can be obtained by adding all the recombinations at region I and the double crossovers and expressing as percentage of the total flies.

% crossovers between *sc* and ec = $[(62 + 88 + 0)/1980] \times 100 = 7.6$ per cent

The percent crossovers at region II (between ec and crossveinless) may be obtained by adding all the single crossovers between ec and crossveinless and adding the double crossovers and determining the percentage of total number of flies as:

% crossovers between ec and cv = $[(89 + 103 + 0)/1980] \times 100 = 9.7$ per cent

Lastly, the distance between *sc* and crossveinless may be obtained as:

% crossovers between *sc* and cv = $[(62 + 88 + 89 + 103 + 0)/1980]$ $\times 100 = 17.3$ percent or by adding the distances between *sc* and ec to ec and cv, i.e. $7.6 + 9.7 = 17.3$ per cent. Now, the distances between the three genes may be given as:

Sc-ec = 7.6%, ec-cv = 9.7 % and *sc*-cv = 17.3 %.

(4) Gene order

The additivity of map distance allows us to place the genes in their linear order. Three linked genes may be in any one of the three different orders, depending upon which gene is in the middle. Suppose that the distance between A–B = 12, B–C = 7 and A–C = 5, then we can determine the correct order as following:

Case I. Assume that A is in the middle, then

B___12___A   A___5___C   B___7___C

In this case, the distance between B and C is not equitable. Therefore, A cannot be in the middle.

Case II. Assume that B is in the middle, then

A___12___B   B___7___C   A___5___C

The distance between A and C is not equitable. Hence, B cannot be in the middle.

Case III. Assume C is in the middle, then

A___5___C   C___7___B

The distance between A and C (5 map units), B and C (7 map units) and between A and B (12 map units) is equitable. Therefore, the gene C must be in the middle and the correct gene order is A-C-B.

CLASS WORK

1. In Drosophila, the mutant known as 'black' b has a black body in contrast to wild type (B), which has grey body. The mutant 'arc' has the wings that are somewhat curved and bent downward, in contrast to the straight wings of the wild type. From the data given below, calculate the crossover value between black and arc.

    B = grey body (wild)   A = straight wings (wild)

    b = black body (mutant)   a = arc wings (mutant)

    Parents: Black body straight wings ×   Grey body arc wings

    Genotypes: bbAA   BBaa

    Gametes: bA   Ba

    F_1 offspring: BbAa

                          (Grey body straight wings)

    Test cross: BbAa   ×   bbaa

                          (Grey body straight wings)   (black body arc wings)

Gametes: BA ab bA Ba   ba

Offspring:	BbAa	Grey body straight wings	=	281
	bbaa	Black body arc wings	=	239
	bbAa	Black body straight wings	=	335
	Bbaa	Gray body arc wings	=	335
		Total		1190

Crossover percentage between black arc = ((No. of black arc + No. of grey straight)/Total no. of flies) × 1190 = ((239 + 281)/1190) = 43.70 per cent.

2. In Drosophila, white eyes (w), forked bristles (f) and miniature wings (m) are sex linked and recessive to the wild-type characters – red eyes (W), straight bristles (F) and long wings (M). In a cross of the females having white eyes (w), forked bristles (f) and miniature wings (m) to wild male and the resultant F_1 females test crossed with white forked miniature males gave the following offspring in a large population.

Phenotype	%
White, forked, miniature	26.8
Red, straight, long	26.8
White, straight, long	13.2
Red, forked, miniature	13.2
White, straight, miniature	6.7
Red, forked, long	6.7
White, forked, long	3.3
Red, straight, miniature	3.3

(a) Designate the non-crossover, single crossover and double crossovers and determine the linkage map.

(b) Determine the percentage of crossover between white and forked, white and miniature and miniature and forked.

Wild form	Mutant form
W = Red eyes	w = White eyes
F = Straight bristles	f = Forked bristles
M = Long wings	m = Miniature wings

$$\frac{\text{w \quad f \quad m}}{\text{w \quad f \quad m}} \; ♀ \; × \; \frac{\text{W \quad F \quad M}}{\quad} \bigg/ \; ♂$$

$$\frac{\text{W \quad F \quad M}}{\text{w \quad f \quad m}} \; ♀ \; × \; \frac{\text{w \quad f \quad m}}{\quad} \bigg/ \; ♂$$

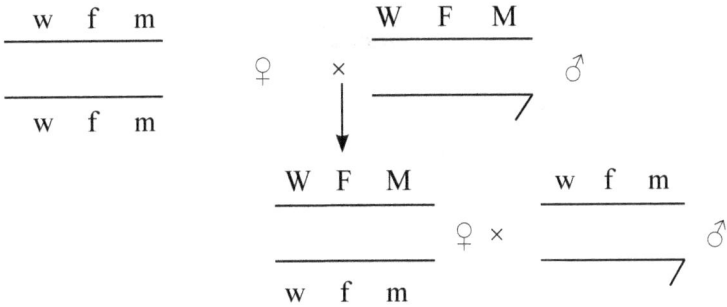

Test cross results:

Genotype	Phenotype	%	Total %	Remarks
W F M / w f m	Red, straight, long	26.8		Parental combinations
w f m / w f m	White, forked, miniature	26.8	53.6	
W f m / w f m	Red, forked, miniature	13.2		Crossovers between W and F (Region-I)
w F M /w f m	White, straight, long	13.2	26.4	
W F m / w f m	Red, straight, miniature	3.3		Crossovers between f and m (Region-II)
w f M / w f m	White, forked, long	3.3	6.6	
W f M / w f m	Red, forked, long	6.7		Double crossovers
w F m / w f m	White, straight, miniature	6.7	13.4	

Distance between white and forked = 26.4% + 13.4% = 39.8%
Distance between forked and miniature = 6.6% + 13.4% = 20.0%
Distance between white and miniature = 39.8% + 20% = 59.8%
The linkage map obtained is:

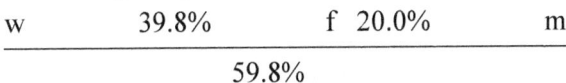

w   39.8%   f   20.0%   m
_____
          59.8%

HOME WORK

5.1.1   What gametes are produced by an individual whose genotype is AB/ab, if crossing over can occur between the genes?

5.1.2   A test cross between AB/ab and ab/ab produced the following offspring:

AB/ab = 180; Ab/ab = 20; aB/ab = 20; ab/ab = 180

Estimate the linkage and recombination percentages.

5.1.3   What gametes are produced by an individual whose genotype is AaBb if the genes are (a) on different chromosomes or (b) on the same chromosomes, assuming no crossing over?

5.1.4   What gametes are produced by male and female Drosophila having the genotypes AB/ab, assuming that crossing over occurs?

5.1.5   A test cross between Ab/aB × ab/ab yielded the progeny in the ratio of 45% Ab/aB, 45% aB/ab, 5% AB/ab and 5% ab/ab. Calculate the chiasma percentage between the two genes.

5.1.6   If the linkage between P and Q genes is 80%, what will be the percentage of crossing over between the two loci?

5.1.7   If the crossover percentages between the genes A and B and B and C are 20% and 10%, respectively, in an individual of ABC/abc genotype, calculate the double crossover percentages of AbC and aBc genotypes.

5.1.8   In a linkage relationship, the distances between a and b and b and c were 10 and 15 map units, respectively. If the coincidence for this portion of the chromosome is 0.6, what kinds of gametes would be expected from an individual of genotypes $a^+ b\ c^+ / a\ b^+ c$? What will be the proportion of each type?

5.1.9   In mice, the genes for frizzy (fr) and albino (c) are linked on a chromosome at a distance of 20 map units. Dihybrid wild-type females in repulsion phase are mated to dihybrid wild-type males in coupling phase. Predict the offspring phenotypic expectations.

5.1.10   Assume that the loci controlling the condition of horns (P for polled and p for horned) and the coat colour (B for black and b for red) are completely linked to each other. Workout the phenotypic ratios expected from crossing of (a) double heterozygous in coupling phase, PB/pb, with a double homozygous recessive, (b) double heterozygous in repulsion phase, Pb/pB, with a double homozygous recessive. (Ans: (a) Polled, black: horned, red: 1:1; (b) Polled, red: horned black ::1:1)

5.1.11   In fruit flies, the allele for black body b is recessive to the allele B for grey body. The allele for vestigial wings v is recessive to the allele V for normal wing-form. A female fly heterozygous for both traits was crossed with a male with black body and vestigial wings. The numbers of progeny of different phenotypes were as follow:

Grey body, normal wings = 252; black body, normal wings = 52; grey body, vestigial wings = 48; black body, vestigial wings = 248.

(a) Assuming the loci to be located on the same chromosome, what is the percentage of crossing over/recombination? (Ans: 16.7%)

(b) Is the linkage in coupling or repulsion phase? (Ans: coupling)

5.1.12   In fruit flies, the allele for black body b is recessive to the allele B for grey body. The allele for vestigial wings v is recessive to the allele V for normal wing-form. Compare the phenotypic outcome from the intercrossing of coupling phase dihybrids with the intercrossing of repulsion phase dihybrids under complete linkage. (Ans: Coupling phase – gray body, normal wings: black body, vestigial wings:: 3:1; repulsion phase – gray body, vestigial wings; gray body, normal wings: black body, normal wings:: 1:2:1)

5.1.13   In Drosophila, the allele for black body b is recessive to the allele B for grey body. The allele for purple eyes p is recessive to the allele P for red eyes. The loci governing these two traits are located on the same chromosome, separated by a distance of 6 map units. A cross is made between double heterozygous Bp/bp and homozygous recessive bp/bp flies. What percentage of the progeny is expected to exhibit black bodies and purple eyes? (Ans: 3%)

5.1.14   A fruit fly of genotype BR/br is test crossed to a fly of br/br genotype. The crossing over between the loci was observed to be 16%. What % of the progeny will be of genotype Bbrr? (Ans: 8%)

5.1.15   In a study of two linked loci, A and B, the test cross AaBb × aabb showed four phenotypic classes in the progeny. Each of the two parental types occurred with a frequency of 46% while each of the other two (crossover type) occurred with a frequency of 4%. How many units of map distance separate these loci? (Ans: 8 map units)

5.1.16   A series of test crosses between three linked loci, D, E and F gave the following crossover frequencies: D and E = 6%; D and F = 22% and e and F = 16%. Draw linkage map. (Ans: D-6-E-16-F)

5.1.17   Three-point test crossing of a triple heterozygote (AaBbCc) with homozygous recessive (aabbcc) for the three loci, based on 1000 progeny, gave the following results.

360 ABC/abc; 90 Abc/abc; 40 ABc/abc; 10 AbC/abc; 360 abc/abc; 90 aBC/abc; 40 abC/abc; 10 aBc/abc

(a) Work out the map distance and linkage relationship between the genes (Ans: A-20-B-10-C)

(b) Work out the coefficient of interference (Ans: 0.0)

5.1.18   In a test cross experiment, the gametes formed by an AaBb individual were found to be AB = 18%, ab = 17%, Ab = 31% and aB = 34%. From this data, (a) find whether the loci A and B are linked or not? (b) If they are linked, what is the map distance between them? (c) If the parents of the AaBb individual were both homozygous, what were their genotypes?

5.1.19   A female Drosophila heterozygous for light eye and vestigial wing (+/lt, +/vg) was crossed with a male homozygous for these alleles (lt vg/lt vg). The phenotypes of the resultant offspring are given below. Calculate the percentage of recombinants.

Wild type = 112; + vg = 16; lt + = 14; lt vg = 108

5.1.20   Consider an organism heterozygous for two genes located on the same chromosome AB/ab. If a single crossover event occurs in the chromosome segment between the two genes in every cell undergoing Meiosis and no multiple crossingover occur in that segment, what will be the recombination frequency between the genes?

5.1.21   In a cross ABD/abd × abd/abd, the most common progeny are ABD/abd and abd/abd, and the least frequent are aBD/abd and Abd/abd. What is the gene order?

5.1.22   Construct a map of a chromosome from the following map distances between individual pairs of genes: r-c 10; c-p 12; p-r 3;

s-c 16; s-r 8. You will discover that the distances are not strictly additive. Why?

5.1.23   The genetic map for three genes is A-8-B-12-D. In a cross ABD/abd × abd/abd, the frequency of aBd is 0.0036. What is the coefficient of coincidence?

5.1.24   Assume the genotype AB/ab is test crossed and produces offspring consisting of 37 A-B-, 11 A-bb, 12 aaB- and 4 aabb. Estimate the percentage recombination between A and B by the square root method.

5.1.25   A laboratory has a homozygous Drosophila line carrying the autosomal recessive genes, a, b and c, linked in that order. Females of this line are crossed with males of a homozygous wild-type line; then, the F_1 heterozygous males with their heterozygous sisters and obtained the following F_2 phenotypes:

1364 +++; 365 a b c; 87 a b +; 84 + + c; 47 a + +; 44 + b c; 5 a + c and 4 + b +.

(a) Estimate the recombination frequencies between a and b; between b and c.

(b) Calculate the coefficient of coincidence.

5.1.26   Three genes on chromosome 9 of corn determine shrunken (sh) versus non-shrunken (Sh) kernels, waxy (wx) versus non-waxy (Wx) and endosperm glossy (gl) versus non-glossy (Gl) leaves. The genetic map of this chromosome region is sh-30-wx-10-gl. From a plant of the genetic constitution Sh wx Gl/sh Wx gl, what is the expected frequency of sh wx gl gametes: (a) in the absence of interference and (b) assuming a coefficient of coincidence of 0.5.

5.1.27   Two dominant mutants in the first linkage group of the guinea pig govern the traits pollex (P_x), which is the activistic return of thumb and little toe, and rough fur (R). When dihybrid pollex, rough pigs (with identical linkage relationships) were crossed to normal pigs, their progeny fell into four phenotypes: 79 rough, 103 normal, 95 rough pollex and 75 pollex. (a) Determine the genotypes of the parents; (b) Calculate the amount of recombination between P_x and R.

5.1.28   In tomatoes, round fruit shape (O) is dominant over elongate (o) and smooth fruit skin (P) is dominant over the peach (p). The

F_1 individuals heterozygous for these pairs of alleles gave the following results.

Smooth, round = 12; Smooth, long = 123; Peach, round = 133; and Peach, long = 12.

Calculate the percent recombination.

5.1.29 Construct a genetic map of the chromosome from the following distances.

r-c = 10 units; c-p = 13 units; p-r = 3 units; s-c = 18 units and s-r = 8 units.

5.1.30 In a cross (ABC)/(abc) × (abc)/(abc), the rarest classes of progeny were (abC)/(abc) and (ABc)/(abc). The parentheses indicate that the order of the genes is unknown. What is the correct sequence of the three genes?

5.1.31 In a dihybrid test cross experiment, the following crossover frequencies were observed.

Jvl-fl = 3%; jvl-e = 13%; fl-e = 11%.

Find out: (a) the gene sequence. (b) How do you account for the fact that the sum of the fl-e and fl-jvl frequencies exceeds the jvl-e frequency?

5.1.32 Assume that genes a and b are linked and show 40% recombination. If a "+ +" individual is crossed with one of "a b", what will be the genotype of the F_1? If the F_1 is crossed with a double recessive, what will be the appearance and genotypes of the offspring?

5.1.33 If the original cross is (+ b) × (a +), what will be the genotype of the F_1? What gametes will it produce? If the F_1 crossed back with the double recessive, what will be the appearance of the offspring?

5.1.34 An individual homozygous for genes c d is crossed with wild type, and the F_1 is crossed back with the double recessive. The appearance of the offspring is:

+ + = 903; c d = 897; + d = 98 and c + = 102

Estimate the strength of linkage between c and d. If assortment between c and d were independent, what should be the result of this cross?

5.1.35 A cross of AA BB/aa bb gave the following segregation in F_2:

AB = 582   Ab = 172   aB = 169   ab = 77

Do you think that a and b are linked or independent? Give

evidence for your answer. Compare the actual distribution with the theoretical expectation on the basis of (1) independent assortment of a and b; (2) 40% crossing over between a and b; (3) 40% crossing over between a and b, using the chi-square test.

5.1.36   In mice, two dominant sex-linked traits are present: *bent* (*Bn*), with a short crooked tail and *tabby* (*Ta*) with dark transverse stripes. Homozygous *bent, tabby* females are mated to normal (wild type) males and all the F_1 offspring are allowed to mate together to produce an F_2. Among 200 F_2 offspring, there were 141 bent and tabby, 47 wild type, 7 tabby, and 5 bent. From these results:

(a) Estimate the amount of recombination between bent and tabby assuming that the male: female ratio is 1:1.

(b) Estimate the amount of recombination when the male: female ratio is variable and unreliable in this colony.

5.1.37   In Drosophila, the mutant known as 'black' b has black body in contrast to the wild type, which has wild type, grey body (B); and the mutant 'arc' has wings that are somewhat curved and bent downward, in contrast to the straight wings of the wild type. If (+ d/+ d) parent is crossed to (c +/ c +) and the resultant F_1 is crossed to double recessive parent, what will be the appearance of F_1 and F_2 and in what proportion?

5.1.38   In fowl, gene S causes silver-coloured plumage; its recessive allele s is responsible for gold. Genes Sl determines slow feathering; its allele sl determines rapid feathering. Both allelic pairs are sex linked. The brown Leghorn male (gold plumage, rapid feathering) were mated with silver-penciled rock female (silver plumage, slow feathering). The F_1 males were mated to females carrying the recessive alleles of both the genes. Identify the crossovers and non-crossovers and map the genes.

	Gold, rapid	Silver, rapid	Gold, slow	Silver, slow
Female	156	28	7	117
Male	127	40	7	94

5.1.39   The curled wings (cu) and spineless bristles (ss) are autosomal recessive traits in Drosophila. The genes responsible for these traits are autosomal, located on chromosome 3. Identify the parents when a wild-type female is crossed with a curled, spineless male and F_2(s) are produced. (Remember that there is no crossing over in male Drosophila). Map the genes.

$$+ + /+ + \qquad \times \qquad cu\ ss\ /\ cu\ ss$$

$$\downarrow$$

F_1 = wild type (+ +/ cu ss)
F_2 = (+ +/ cu ss) ♀ × (+ +/ cu ss) ♂

$$\downarrow$$

F_2 offspring:

	+ +	cu ss	Phenotype	No. of flies
+ +	+ +/+ +	+ +/ cu ss	Wild type	292
+ ss	+ +/+ ss	+ ss / cu ss	Normal, spineless	7
cu +	+ +/ cu +	cu +/ cu ss	Curled, normal	9
cu ss	+ +/ cu ss	cu ss / cu ss	Curled, spineless	92

5.1.40 Assume that genes a and b are linked and show 40 per cent of recombination. If a + +/+ + individual is crossed with one that is a b/ a b, what will be the genotype of the F_1? What gametes will the F_1 produce, and in what proportions? If the F_1 is crossed with a double recessive, what will be the appearance and genotypes of the offspring?

If a cross is made between + b/+ b × a +/a +, what will be the genotype of the F_1? What gametes will it produce? If the F_1 is crossed back to a double recessive, what will be the appearance of the offspring and appearance of the offspring of F_2 (F_1 × F_1)?

5.1.41 An individual homozygous for genes c d is crossed with wild type, and the F_1 is crossed back with the double recessive. The appearance of the offspring is as follows:

903	+	+
897	c	d
98	+	d
102	c	+

Estimate the strength of linkage between c and d. If the assortment between c and d were independent, what would be the result of this cross? If a cross is made between homozygous + d individual and a homozygous c + one, what would be the result of the cross of F_1 with the double recessive?

5.1.42 In Drosophila, the mutant known as "black" b has a black body in contrast to the wild type that has a gray body, and the mutant "arc" a has wings that are somewhat curved and bent downward, in contrast to the straight wings of the wild type. From the data given below, calculate the crossover value between black and arc.

(a) Black straight × gray arc; F_1 ♀ × black arc ♂ produced the following offspring:

Gray straight	281
Gray arc	335
Black straight	335
Black arc	239

(b) Black arc × wild type; F_1 ♀ crossed with black arc ♂ produced the offspring:

Gray straight	1641
Gray arc	1251
Black straight	1180
Black arc	1532

5.1.43 In Drosophila, the mutant known as black (*b*) has a black body in contrast to the wild type, which has a gray body (*B*); and the mutant vestigial (*vg*) has short wings, in contrast to the normal wings (*Vg*) of the wild type. From the data given below, calculate the crossover value between black and vestigial.

(a) Black vestigial × wild type (gray normal) F_1 ♀ × black vestigial ♂ produced the following offspring:

Gray body normal wings	822
Gray body vestigial wings	130
Black body normal wings	161
Black body vestigial wings	652

(b) Black normal × Gray vestigial F_1 ♀ × black vestigial ♂ produced the following offspring:

Gray body normal wings	283
Gray body vestigial wings	1294
Black body normal wings	1418
Black body vestigial wings	241

Calculate the crossover value between black and vestigial.

(c) The cross heterozygous wild-type female × black body vestigial wings male produced following progeny:

Gray body normal wings	140
Gray body vestigial wings	39
Black body normal wings	42
Black body vestigial wings	147

Does this data indicate linkage between genes for body colour and wing length? What is the frequency of recombination? Show the arrangement of these genetic markers on a chromosome diagrammatically.

(d) The cross heterozygous wild type female × black body vestigial wings male produced following progeny:

Gray body normal wings	15
Gray body vestigial wings	200
Black body normal wings	225
Black body vestigial wings	11

Does this data indicate linkage between genes for body colour and wing length? What is the frequency of recombination? Show the arrangement of these genetic markers on a chromosome diagrammatically.

5.1.44 In rats, dark eyes are due to the interaction of two genes R and P, the recessive allele of either producing light eyes. These genes are located on the same chromosome. When homozygous dark eyed rats, $+ +/ + +$ were crossed with double recessive ones, r p/r p and the F_1 crossed back with the double recessives gave 1255 dark eyed and 1777 light eyed offspring. When $+ p/+ p$ animals were crossed with $r +/r +$ ones and the F_1 crossed back with the double recessive, the offspring produced were 174 dark eyed and 1540 light eyed. Calculate the crossover value between r and p.

5.1.45 In Drosophila, white eye colour and club wing are both sex linked with a crossover value of about 15 percent. If a wild-type female (red long) is crossed with a white club male, what will be the appearance of the offspring? If both males and females of the F_1 are crossed back to pure white club stock, what will be the offspring in each case?

5.1.46 In fowl, assume that e (early feathering) and B (barring) are sex linked and show 20% crossing over (in the male only). If a male from a cross of late feathered barred male × early black female is mated with an early black female, what will be the appearance of their offspring as to feathering and barring?

5.1.47 Assume that genes a and b are linked, with a crossover percentage of 20 and that c and d are also linked with a crossover percentage of 10, but are in another chromosome. Cross a plant homozygous for AB CD with one that is ab cd and cross the F_1 back on ab cd. What will be the appearance of the offspring of this cross?

5.1.48 In Drosophila, assume that three pairs of alleles +/+, +/y and +/z, each mutant gene is recessive to its wild-type allele. A cross between females heterozygous at these three loci and wild-type males gave the following results. Find out the sequence of the linked genes in their chromosomes. Calculate the map distance between the genes and the coefficient of coincidence.

Males:	+ + +	=	1010
Females:	+ + +	=	30
	+ + z	=	32
	+ y +	=	441
	+ y z	=	1
	x + +	=	0
	x + z	=	430
	x y +	=	27
	x y z	=	39

(Ans: x–y = 6; y–z = 7; x–z = 13; coincidence = 0.2364)

From the data given below, calculate the crossover value between black and grey:

(a) Black straight × grey arc; F_1 ♀ × black arc ♂ gives: 21 Grey straight, 335 Grey arc, 335 Black straight and 239 Black arc offspring.

(b) Black arc × wild type; F_1 ♀ × black arc ♂ gives: 1641 Grey straight, 1251 Grey arc, 1180 Black straight and 1532 Black arc offspring.

5.1.49 There are two pairs of alleles in tomatoes: Cu, "curl" (leaves curled); cu, normal leaves; Bk, "beakless" fruits; and bk, "beaked" fruits, having sharp-pointed protuberance on blossom end of the mature fruit. The cross of two doubly heterozygous "curl beakless" plants yields four phenotypic classes in the offspring, of which 23.04 are "normal beaked". Find out whether these two pairs of genes linked. How do you know?

5.1.50   The cross $+ + +/$ a b c ($♀$) $×$ a b c $/$ a b c ($♂$) Drosophila flies gave the following test cross results. Estimate the coincidence.

a–b single crossovers = 5.75%; b–c single crossovers = 8.08%; a–c double crossovers = 0.25%

5.1.51   A cross was made between yellow, bar, vermilion female flies and wild males and the F_1 females were crossed with y B v males. The following results were obtained when 1000 progeny were counted.

Y B v and $+ + +$	546
Y $+ +$ and $+ $B v	244
Y $+$ v and $+$ B $+$	160
Y B $+$ and $+ +$ v	50

Determine the order in which the three loci occur in the chromosome(s) and prepare a chromosome map.

5.1.52   Map the genes based on the following two-point test cross recombination data.

Gene loci	% recombination	Gene loci	% recombination
a, b	50	b, d	13
a, c	15	b, e	50
a, d	38	c, d	50
a, e	8	c, e	7
b, c	50	d, e	45

5.1.53   An inbred strain of snapdragons with violet flowers and dull leaves was crossed to another inbred strain with white flowers and shiny leaves. The F_1 plants, which all had violet flowers and dull leaves, were backcrossed to the strain with white flowers and shiny leaves and the following F_2 plants were obtained: 50 violet, dull; 46 white, shiny; 12 violet, shiny; and 10 white, dull.

(a) Which of the four classes in the F_2 are recombinants?

(b) What is the evidence that the genes for flower colour and leaf texture are linked?

(c) Diagram the crosses of this experiment.

(d) What is the frequency of recombination between the flower colour and leaf texture genes?

(e) What is the genetic map distance between these genes?

5.1.54 The Drosophila females heterozygous for three recessive X-linked markers, y (yellow body), ct (cut wings) and m (miniature wings) and their wild-type alleles were crossed to y ct m males. The following progeny were obtained:

Phenotype	No. of flies
Yellow, cut, miniature	30
Wild type	33
Yellow	10
Cut, miniature	12
Miniature	8
Yellow, cut	5
Yellow, miniature	1
Cut	1
Total	100

(a) What classes are parental types?

(b) Which classes represent double crossovers?

(c) Which gene is in the middle of the other two?

(d) What was the genotype of the heterozygous females used in the cross? Show the correct linkage phase and the correct order of the markers along the chromosomes.

5.1.55 Singed bristles (sn), crossveinless wings (cv) and vermilion eye colour (v) are due to recessive mutant alleles of three X-linked genes in Drosophila melanogaster. When a female heterozygous for each of the three genes was test crossed with a singed, crossveinless, vermilion male, the following progeny were obtained:

Phenotype	No. of flies
Singed, crossveinless, vermilion	3
Crossveinless, vermilion	392
Vermilion	34
Crossveinless	61
Singed, crossveinless	32
Singed, vermilion	65
Singed	410
Wild type	3
Total	1000

Find out the order of these three genes on the X-chromosome. What are the genetic map distances between *sn* and *cv*, *sn* and *v*, and *cv* and *v*? What is the coefficient of coincidence? (Ans: cv-7.2-sn-13.2-v. Distance between cv and v is 7.2 + 13.2 = 20.4 cM. Coincidence = 0.63).

5.1.56   A woman has two dominant traits, each caused by a mutation in a different gene: cataract (an eye abnormality), which she inherited from her father, and polydactyly (an extra finger), which she inherited from her mother. Her husband has neither of the traits. If the genes for these two traits are 15 cM apart on the same chromosome, what is the chance that the first child of this couple will have both cataract and polydactyly?

(Ans: To calculate the chance that the child will have both traits, we first need to determine the linkage phase of the mutant alleles in the woman's genotype. Because she inherited the cataract mutation from her father and the polydactyly mutation from her mother, the mutant alleles must be on opposite chromosomes, i.e. in the repulsion linkage phase: C +/+ P. For a child to inherit both mutant alleles, the woman would have to produce an egg that carried a recombinant chromosome, C P. We can estimate the probability of this event from the distance between the two genes, 15 cM, which, because of interference, should be equivalent to 15 percent recombination. However, only half the recombinants will be C P. Thus, chance that the child will inherit both mutant alleles is 15/2 = 7.5 percent.)

5.1.57 The Drosophila females heterozygous for three recessive mutations, a, b and c, were crossed to males homozygous for all three mutations. The cross yielded the following results:

Phenotype	No. of flies
+ + +	75
+ + c	348
+ b c	96
a + +	110
a b +	306
a b c	65

Construct a linkage map showing the correct order of these genes and estimate the distances between them.

5.1.58 The female *Drosophila* heterozygous for three recessive mutations *e* (*ebony* body), *st* (*scarlet* eyes) and *ss* (*spineless* bristles) were test crossed and the following progeny were obtained:

Phenotype	No. of flies
Wild-type	67
Ebony	8
Ebony, scarlet	68
Ebony, spineless	347
Ebony, scarlet, spineless	78
Scarlet	368
Scarlet, spineless	10
Spineless	54

(a) What indicates that the genes are linked?

(b) What was the genotype of the original heterozygous females?

(c) What is the order of the genes?

(d) What is the map distance between *e* and *st*?

(e) What is the map distance between *e* and *ss*?

(f) What is the coefficient of coincidence?

(g) Diagram the crosses in this experiment.

5.1.59 The female Drosophila flies homozygous for three X-linked mutations: y, yellow body; B, bar eye shape; v, vermilion eye colour were mated to wild-type males. The F_1 females, which had gray bodies and bar eyes with dark red pigment, were then crossed to y B+ v males, yielding the following results:

Phenotype	No. of flies
Yellow, bar, vermilion Wild-type	581
Yellow Bar, vermilion	200
Yellow, vermilion Bar	173
Yellow, bar Vermilion	46

Determine the order of these three loci on the X-chromosome and estimate the distances between them.

5.1.60 In Drosophila, there are three genes, x, y and z, with each mutant allele recessive to the wild-type allele. A cross between females heterozygous for these three loci and wild-type males yielded the following progeny:

	Phenotype	No. of flies
Females	+ + +	1515
Males	+ + +	55
	+ + z	630
	+ y z	65
	x + +	43
	x y +	640
	x y z	52
	Total:	3000

Using these data, construct a linkage map of the three genes and calculate the coefficient of coincidence.

5.1.61 In Drosophila, a kidney-bean shaped eye is produced by a recessive gene on the third chromosome. Orange eye colour called "*cardinal*" is produced by the recessive gene *cd* on the same chromosome. Between these two loci is a third locus with a recessive allele e, producing *ebony* body colour. Homozygous kidney, cardinal females are mated to homozygous ebony males. The trihybrid F_1 females are then test crossed to produce the F_2. Among the 4000 F_2 progeny the following were found:

Phenotype	No. of flies	Phenotype	No. of flies
Kidney, cardinal	1761	Kidney	97
Ebony	1773	Ebony, cardinal	89
Kidney, ebony	128	Kidney, ebony, cardinal	6
Cardinal	138	Wild type	8

(a) Determine the linkage relationships in the parents and F_1 trihybrids.

(b) Measure the map distances.

5.1.62 The following four pairs of genes are linked on chromosome 2 of a plant.

Aw and *aw* = purple and green stems

O and *o* = oval and spherical fruit

Wo and *wo* = wooly and smooth leaves

Dil and *dil* = normal and diluted leaf colour

The crossover frequencies among the above genes were found to be:

Wo-o = 14%; *wo-dil* = 9%; *wo-aw* = 20%; *dil-o* = 6%; *dil-aw* = 12%; *o-aw* = 7%.

(a) What is the order of genes on chromosome 2?

(b) Why is not the *wo-aw* two-pair crossover frequency greater?

5.1.63 In tomatoes, the mutant genes o (oblate = flattened fruit), p (peach = hairy fruit) and s (compound inflorescence = many flowers in a cluster) were found to be on chromosome 2. From the following data on test cross mating of an F_1 heterozygote for all three genes × homozygous recessive for all three genes, determine:

(a) The sequence of these three genes in chromosome 2

(b) The genotypes of the homozygous parents used in making the F_1 heterozygote

(c) The recombination distance between the genes

(d) The coefficient of coincidence

Phenotypes of test cross progeny	No. of plants
+ + +	73
+ + s	348
+ p +	2
+ p s	96
o + +	110
o + s	2
o p +	306
o p s	63

5.1.64 In Drosophila, the following results of trihybrid test cross were obtained. Construct a genetic map.

Phenotypes of test cross progeny	No. of flies
+ m +	218
w + f	236
+ + f	168
w m +	178
+ m f	95
w + +	101
+ + +	3
w m f	1

51.65 In Drosophila, the mutant type alleles are *sc* (scute, or loss of certain thoracic bristles), ec (echinus or roughened eye surface) and vg. A cross of *sc* ec vg flies with homozygous wild type and then test cross the F₁ females (*sc*/+ ec/+ vg/+) gave the following offspring. Determine the order in which the loci occur in the chromosome and prepare a chromosome map.

Phenotypes of test cross progeny	No. of Flies
sc ec vg	235
+ + +	241
sc ec +	243
+ + vg	233
sc + vg	12
+ ec +	14
sc + +	14
+ ec vg	16

5.1.66 (a) In a test cross of + b +/a + c Drosophila females mated with a b c male, the following offspring were produced:

+ b +/a b c	358
a b +/a b c	46
a b c/a b c	4
+ b c/a b c	98
a + +/a b c	92
a + c/a b c	352
+ + +/a b c	6
+ + c/a b c	44

Calculate the percentage of recombinants and construct the linkage map.

(b) In another cross, the female flies heterozygous for three recessive mutations, a, b and c, were crossed to males homozygous for all three mutations. The cross yielded the following results.

+ + +	225
+ + c	1044
+ b c	288
a + +	330
a b +	918
a b c	195

Construct the linkage map showing the distances between a b c and show the correct order.

5.1.67   A cross was made between the Drosophila flies containing the homozygous alleles for scute (*sc*), echinus (*ec*) and crossveinless (*cv*) with homozygous wild type (normal) to get *sc ec cv*/ + + + females, which were then test crossed to obtain the following test cross progeny. Map the order in which three loci occur in the chromosome and prepare a chromosome map.

sc ec cv	417
+ + +	430
sc + +	25
+ ec cv	29
sc ec +	44
+ + cv	37
Total	982

5.1.68   In Drosophila, the allele B for grey body is dominant to the allele b for black body. Another locus controls the wing shape; the allele for straight wing C is dominant to the allele for curved wing c. The loci controlling these traits are linked. A gray-bodied, straight-winged fly, homozygous for both the traits was mated with a black-bodied, curved wing fly. An F_1 female obtained from the above cross was then test crossed with a male having a black body and curved wing. (a) Identify the phenotypes expected among the test cross progeny if there is no crossing over. (b) Identify the phenotypes expected among the test cross progeny if there is some crossing over between these two loci. Would you expect the progeny phenotypes obtained from this mating to occur in equal frequencies? Explain why or why not.

5.1.69   In mice, the allele C for normal tail is dominant to the allele c for crinky tail. Another locus controls the coat type; the allele for normal coat S is dominant to the allele for soft coat s. A mouse with crinky tail and soft coat was crossed to a true-breeding normal-tail and normal-coat mouse. All the F_1 offspring had normal tail and normal coat. The F_1 mice was test crossed and the results obtained in the progeny were: crinky tail, soft coat = 104; crinky tail, normal = 103; normal tail, normal coat = 97; normal tail and soft coat = 100. Conduct a chi-square test to determine if the two genes are linked.

5.1.70   In fruit flies, the allele for black body b is recessive to the allele B for grey body. The allele for vestigial wings v is recessive to the allele V for normal wing form. A female fruit fly heterozygous for both traits was crossed with a male with black body and vestigial wings. The progeny phenotypes and their numbers were as follows:

Grey body, normal wings = 252; Black body, normal wings = 52

Grey body, vestigial wings = 48; Black body, vestigial wings = 248

Do the results of this test cross support the hypothesis that the genes for these two traits are linked? Explain.

If these loci are linked, what is the percentage of crossing/recombination?

5.1.71   Test crossing of double heterozygotes in coupling phase (AB/ab) with a double recessive (ab/ab) yielded 44% AaBb; 44% aabb (both these are parental classes) and 6% Aabb; 6% aaBb (both these are recombinant classes). Calculate the map distance between the two loci.

5.1.72   Feather morphology (normal versus frizzled) in chickens is controlled by a single autosomal locus with two alleles; the allele for frizzled feather F is dominant to the allele for normal feather condition f. Another locus controls plumage colour; white plumage is caused by the dominant allele I and the coloured plumage by its recessive allele i. A double heterozygote female (frizzled white) was test crossed to a double homozygous (normal, coloured) male and gave the following data in the progeny:

Frizzled white = 45; Frizzled coloured = 7; normal white = 12; normal coloured = 36.

Work out the map distance between the two loci.

Work out the linkage relationship of the genes in the F_1 and the genotype of the parents of the F_1 individual.

5.1.73   Two-point test crosses were made for determining the distance between three loci, viz. A, B and C. Examination of the 400 test cross progeny gave the following data.

Test cross I: A and B parental = 352 and crossover = 48

Test cross II: A and C parental = 376 and crossover = 24

Find out the distance between three loci.

Can the order of genes be determined from this information? Explain.

5.1.74   In Drosophila, the cinnabar (cn) eye, curved wings (c) and plexus wings (px) are mutants to their wild normal eye (Cn), straight wings (C) and non-plexus wings (Px). The number of flies obtained by test crossing the F_1 wild females with the cinnabar eye, curved wings and plexus wings are given below. Calculate the genetic distances and prepare a linkage map.

Phenotype	Genotype	No. of flies	Total	Remarks
Wild	+ + + / cn c px	329		
Cinnabar, curved, plexus	cn c px / cn c px	296	625	Parental combinations
Cinnabar	cn + + / cn c px	119		
Curved, Plexus	+ c px / cn c px	86	205	Crossovers at region I
Plexus	+ + px / cn c px	82		
Cinnabar, curved	cn c + / cn c px	63	145	Crossovers at region II
Curved	+ c + / cn c px	15		
Cinnabar, plexus	cn + px / cn c px	10	25	Double crossovers
Total		1000	1000	

5.1.75   Three two-point test crosses were made among loci A, B and C, and crossover frequencies were calculated as follows: A and C = 16%; A and B = 35%; B and C = 19%. Prepare a chromosome map showing the relative positions and the distances between the three loci.

5.1.76   In Drosophila, the allele for grey body colour B is dominant to allele for black body b; the allele for red eye colour P is dominant to allele for purple eye p; the allele for normal wings V is dominant to vestigial wings v. Two true-breeding strains having contrasting phenotypes are crossed to produce F_1 individuals that are heterozygous for the three loci. In the F_1 heterozygotes, all the dominant genes are located on one chromosome; all the recessive alleles are on the other homologous chromosome (coupling phase linkage). The F_1 females heterozygous for each of the three loci BbPpVv are mated to male flies that are homozygous recessive for each of the loci bbppvv. The 1000 progeny obtained from the cross fell into the eight phenotypic classes listed below.

Body colour	Phenotype of		No. of offspring
	Eye colour	Wing shape	
Grey	Red	Normal	410
Black	Purple	Vestigial	411
Grey	Purple	Vestigial	29
Black	Red	Normal	28
Grey	Red	Vestigial	60
Black	Purple	Normal	59
Grey	Purple	Normal	2
Black	Red	Vestigial	1

Construct a linkage map. Calculate the percentage of interference and coincidence.

5.1.77 The results obtained from a test cross experiment on a line of Drosophila flies are given below. The mutant recessive genes are crossveinless (cv, absence of cross veins in the wings), echinus (ec, missing bristles on the body) and cut wing (ct, cut wing). Construct a linkage map and draw your conclusions. F_1 genotype: (+ cv +/ec + ct) × ec cv ct males

Phenotype	Genotype	No. of flies	Total	Remarks
Crossveinless	+ cv +	2207		
Echinus, cut	ec + ct	2125	4332	Parental combinations
Echinus crossveinless	ec cv +	273		
Cut	+ + ct	265	538	Crossovers at region I
Echinus	ec + +	217		
Crossveinless, cut	+ cv ct	223	440	Crossovers at region II
Wild type	+ + +	5		
Echinus, crossveinless, cut	ec cv ct	3	8	Double crossovers
Total		5318	5318	

(Ans: ec-cv = 10.1 + 0.1 = 10.2%; cv-ct = 8.3 + 0.1 = 8.4%; ec and
ct = 10.1 + 8.3 + 0.2 = 18.6%)

5.1.78 In corn, the F_1 plants from the cross of coloured, shrunken, starchy
× colourless, full, waxy were crossed with colourless, shrunken,
waxy plants and the following progeny were observed. Map the
positions of c (coloured), s (shrunken) and w (waxy) genes and
estimate the coincidence.

Phenotype	No. of plants
Coloured, shrunken, starchy	2538
Colourless, full, waxy	2708
Coloured, full, waxy	116
Colourless, shrunken, starchy	113
Coloured, shrunken, waxy	601
Colourless, full, starchy	626
Coloured, full, starchy	4
Colourless, shrunken, waxy	2
Total	5318

(Ans: c-s = 3.50; s-w = 18.38; c-w = 21.88; coincidence = 0.13)

5.1.79 In Drosophila, yellow body is sex linked and recessive to the
gray body of the wild fly. Vermilion eye is also sex linked and
recessive to the wild red eye. The genes for yellow and vermilion
show about 28% crossing over. The gene for vestigial wings is
in one of the autosomes. If a homozygous yellow-bodied, red-
eyed, long-winged female is crossed with a homozygous gray-
bodied, vermilion-eyed, vestigial-winged male and if an F_1 female
is crossed with a yellow, vermilion, vestigial male, what will be
the proportions in the offspring of this last cross?

5.1.80 In sweet peas, a cross of a homozygous procumbent, hairy,
white-flowered plant with a bush, glabrous, coloured-flowered
one produces an F_1, that is all procumbent, hairy and coloured
flowered. If this F_1 is crossed on a bush, glabrous, white-flowered
plant, the offspring would be expected to show approximately
the following distribution. Map the genes and also calculate the
coefficient of coincidence and interference.

Procumbent, hairy, coloured	6%
Procumbent, hairy, white	19%

Procumbent, glabrous, coloured	6%
Procumbent, glabrous, white	19%
Bush, hairy, coloured	19%
Bush, hairy, white	6%
Bush, glabrous, coloured	19%
Bush, glabrous, white	6%

5.1.81 In Drosophila, white eyes (w), miniature wings (m) and forked bristles (f) are sex linked and recessive to the wild-type characters: red eyes, long wings and straight bristles. In a cross of wfm/wfm × + + +, the F₁ females cross with w f m males gave the following in a large population:

Phenotype	Per cent
White, forked, miniature	26.8
Red, straight, long	26.8
White, straight, long	13.2
Red, forked, miniature	13.2
White, straight, miniature	6.7
Red, forked, long	6.7
White, forked, long	3.3
Red, straight, miniature	3.3

Designate the non-crossover, single crossover and double crossover classes.

Determine the percentage of crossing over between white and forked, white and miniature, and miniature and forked, and from this determine the order of these genes in the chromosome.

Construct a chromosome map of the genes.

5.1.82 In Drosophila, the mutant "morula" (m) causes the eye facets to be irregular in size, shape and colour than those of normal eye; mutant "arc" (a) causes the wings to somewhat bent downwards, in contrast to normal straight wings and the mutant "black" (b) causes black body in contrast to the wild grey body. The number of various types of flies resulting from four back cross experiments are given below. In each of the experiments, determine the crossover percentage between black and arc, arc and morula and black and morula. Map the chromosome for these three points.

Cross I: Arc, black, morula × wild type; F_1 ♀ × arc, black, morula ♂
Cross II: Arc, black × morula; F_1 ♀ × arc, black, morula ♂
Cross III: Black, morula × arc; F_1 ♀ × arc, black, morula ♂
Cross IV: Black × arc, morula; F_1 ♀ × arc, black, morula ♂

	Cross I	Cross II	Cross III	Cross IV
Wild type	95	164	613	3
Black	40	187	445	13
Arc	713	21	38	113
Morula	851	7	82	107
Arc black	884	8	55	96
Black morula	666	15	29	120
Arc morula	33	187	467	14
Arc black morula	79	133	514	2

5.1.83   In rats, dark eyes are due to the interaction of two genes R and P, the recessive allele of either producing light eyes. These genes are on the same chromosome. RRpp animals have pink eyes and light-coloured coats; rrPP animals have red eyes and light-coloured coats. RR PP animals have dark eyes and dark coats. Albinism cc (pink eyes and white coat) is also linked with r and p. ccrr, ccR(r), ccpp, ccP(p) are albino and have colourless eyes at birth. Design an experiment to measure this linkage and to map the chromosome containing r, p and c, giving all the necessary steps and crosses.

5.1.84   In Drosophila, three linked genes a, b and c gave the following results when a c females were crossed to b males and the F_1 inbred (F_1 females +, F_1 males a c).

F_2 phenotypes	No. of females	No. of males
a	49	2
b	0	428
c	49	48
+	451	23
a b	0	47
a c	451	428
b c	0	1
a b c	0	23

Are the three genes sex linked or autosomal? Determine the genotype of parents and offspring and gene order. What is recombination percent between the three genes? What is the coefficient of coincidence and is there any interference?

5.1.85 A homozygous Drosophila line carry the autosomal recessive genes a, b and c linked in that order. Females of this line are crossed with males of a homozygous wild-type line. Then, F_1 heterozygous males are crossed with their heterozygous sisters and obtained the following F_2 phenotypes: 1364 + + +, 365 a b c, 87 a b +, 84 + + c, 47 a + +, 44 + b c, 5 a + c and 4 + b +.

What is the recombinant frequency between a and b? between b and c?

What is the coefficient of coincidence?

5.1.86 In tomatoes, round fruit shape (O) is dominant over elongate (o), and the smooth fruit skin (P) is dominant over peach (p). Test crosses of F_1 individuals heterozygous for these pairs of alleles gave the following results.

Smooth, round = 24; smooth, long = 246; peach, round = 266; peach, long = 42

In the F_2, were the two pairs of alleles linked in the coupling or repulsion phase? Calculate the percentage of recombination.

5.1.87 In fowls, the gene S determines silver-coloured plumage; its recessive allele s determines gold. Gene Sl determines slow feathering; its allele sl determines rapid feathering. Both allelic pairs are sex linked. Brown Leghorn males (gold plumage, rapid feathering) are crossed with silver-penciled rock females (silver plumage, slow feathering) and F_1 males mated to females carrying the recessive alleles of both genes. Among the progeny of this crosses were:

	Gold, rapid	Silver, rapid	Gold, slow	Silver, slow
Females	312	56	14	234
Males	254	80	14	188

Diagram the crosses, designate the crossover and non-crossover types among the test cross progeny. What is the percentage of recombination?

5.1.88 In Drosophila, assume that there are three pairs of alleles +/x, +/y and +/z. Each mutant gene is recessive to its wild-type allele. A cross between females heterozygous at these three loci and wild-type male gave the following results.

Females	+ + +	2020
Males	+ + +	60
	+ + z	64
	+ y +	882
	+ y z	2
	x + +	0
	x + z	860
	x y +	54
	x y z	78

What is the sequence of these linked genes in their chromosome? Calculate the map distances between the genes and the coefficient of coincidence.

5.1.89 Assume that in Drosophila there are three pairs of alleles +/n, +/o and +/p. Genes n, o and p are all recessives and sex linked. They occur in the order n-o-p in the X-chromosome, with n being 12 map units from o and o being 10 units from p. The coefficient of coincidence for this region of the X-chromosome is 0.5. From a cross between females of the genotype $+ + p / n o +$ and wild-type male, predict the kinds and frequencies of phenotypes that would be expected to occur in a progeny of 2000 individuals.

5.1.90 In a series of experiments in Drosophila beginning with a mating between *dachs* (d) males and *black* (*b*) females in F_2, there were 186 wild type, 71 *dachs*, 93 *black* and 0 *dachs*, *black*. Do these results indicate that the loci of genes d and b are very closely linked? Explain your answer.

5.1.91 In Drosophila, the curled wings (cu) and spineless bristles (ss) are autosomal recessive characters. The genes giving rise to these characters are located on chromosome 3. Beginning with a wild-type female and a curled, spineless male, prepare a diagram showing parents and progenies through an F_2 generation. Suppose in the F_2 generation the number of various kinds of flies obtained were: 292 wild, 9 curled, 92 curled, spineless and 7 spineless, estimate the map distance between *cu* and *ss*. Explain your method and calculate the distance.

5.1.92 The following diagram shows a linkage map of three genes a, b and c, where the distances are given in centimorgans (map units).

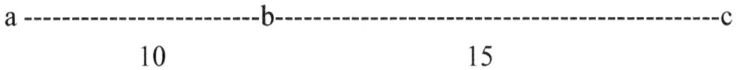

a ----------------------b--c

         10   15

Assume the coefficient of coincidence to be 0.40. Among 1000 gametes from an individual of genotype A B C/a b c, what are the expected numbers of each of the possible allele combinations?

(Ans: Since we know the frequencies of recombination (0.10 and 0.15) and also that the coefficient of coincidence equals 0.40, we can write the frequency of double crossovers that should be observed as $0.40 \times 0.10 \times 0.15 = 0.006$. These are of two types: A b C and a B c, and so the expected number among 1000 gametes is 3 of each. In the a-b interval, the expected proportion of single recombinants equals $0.10 - 0.006 = 0.094$. The trick here is to remember to subtract the double crossovers. There are two types of single crossovers in this interval A b c and a B C and among 1000 gametes, the expected number of each is $94/2 = 47$. Similarly, in b-c interval, the expected proportion of single recombinants equals $0.15 - 0.006 = 0.144$. In this case the two types are A B c and a B C and each has an expected number of $144/1 = 72$. The remaining gametes of which there are $1000 - 6 - 94 - 144 = 756$ m are expected to be divided equally between the non-recombinant A B C and a b c types, for an expected number of $756/2 = 378$ each).

5.1.93 In a plant-breeding experiment, the individual plants homozygous for various combinations of linked genes R and T, i.e., RR TT, RR tt, rr TT and rr tt were crossed to produce F_1 plants, which were then self-fertilized to produce an F_2 generation. R is dominant to r and T is dominant to t. What is the chromosomal constitution for each F_1 parent of the following F_2 phenotypic distributions?

	Self-fertilized F_1 plants		F_2 phenotypes	
	R T	R t	r T	r t
(a)	106	34	0	0
(b)	0	0	104	36
(c)	99	0	31	0
d)	64	10	8	18

5.1.94 A cross was made between the homozygous genotypes A B C and a b c. The triple heterozygous F_1 offspring were then crossed with homozygous a b c. The resulting progeny and their numbers were:

A B C / a b c	177
A B c / a b c	89
A b C / a b c	81
A b c / a b c	180
a B C / a b c	173
a B c / a b c	71
a b C / a b c	68
A b c / a b c	161
Total	1000

5.1.95 The following data show 1000 gametes obtained from a triply heterozygous parent in a three-point test cross to determine the genetic map of three linked genes. Neither the parental genotype of the heterozygous parent nor the order of the genes is known.

Gamete	Number of gametes
F G H	4
F G h	41
F g H	393
F g h	50
f G H	64
f G h	413
f g H	33
f g h	2

(a) What is the genotype of the heterozygous parent?

(b) What is the correct linear order of the genes?

(c) What is the map distance between middle gene and its nearest neighbor?

(d) What is the map distance between middle gene and its farthest neighbors?

(e) What is the expected number of double crossovers?

(f) What is the coincidence and the interference?

Answer:

(a) The most frequent classes of the progeny imply that the genotype of the heterozygous parent is F g H/f G h, with the gene order still to be determined.

(b) Comparison of the parental classes with the double-recombinants (least common) identifies the gene in the middle, which is G in this case. Thus, the correct linear order of the genes is F G H or H G F.

(c) The map distance between F and G is $(74 + 6)/1000 = 0.08$. The map distance between G and H is $(114 + 6)/1000 = 0.12$. Hence the map distance between middle gene G and its nearest neighbor F is $0.08 = 8\%$ map units $= 8$ cM.

(d) The map distance between the middle gene G and its farthest neighbor H is $0.12 = 12\% = 12$ map units $= 12$ cM.

(e) The expected number of double crossovers is the product of the frequencies of recombination in each region and the total number of progeny: $0.08 \times 0.12 \times 1000 = 9.6$

(f) The coincidence c is the observed number of double crossovers over the expected or $6/9.6 = 0.625$. The interference $i = (1 - c) = 1 - 0.625 = 0.375$.

5.1.96 A strain of guinea pigs is homozygous for some alleles of five genes AA bb cc DD ee. A second strain is the genotype aa BB CC dd EE. The genes D and E are linked and 20 cM apart. All other genes assort independently. The two strains are crossed to generate F_1 individuals and the F_1 females are test crossed. (a) Considering only the genes A, B and C, what is the probability of obtaining an offspring from the test cross that has the same phenotype as the F_1 female parent?

Considering all the genes, what is the probability that an offspring from the test cross has the same phenotype as the F_1 female parent?

5.1.97 In mice, short-ear and dilution show almost complete linkage. Assuming no crossovers,   what is the expected result in F_2 if (a) a short-eared (DDss) and a dilute (ddSS) mouse are crossed; (b) what results in F_1? (c) What results in F_1 and F_2 if the cross is DDSS × ddss? (d) Which cross shows coupling and which is repulsion? (e) Is there any real difference between F_1 mice resulting from the two crosses?

5.1.98   In rabbits, the gene C is responsible for coloured fur in contrast to its recessive allele causing the body to be colourless (albino). Another allele determines whether the fur colour is black (B) or brown (b). A homozygous brown rabbits were crossed with homozygous albinos. The F_1s were then crossed to homozygous double recessive rabbits, producing the progeny types: black 21, brown 58, albino 98. Are the genes *b* and *c* linked? Estimate the frequency of recombination. Illustrate through a diagram showing the arrangement of these markers on the chromosomes.

5.1.99   In tomatoes, tall vine (D) is dominant over the dwarf (d) and spherical fruit shape (P) is dominant over pear shape (p). The genes for these two traits, i.e. vine height and fruit shape are linked with a recombination percentage of 30.0. One tall plant (Cross-I) with spherical fruit was crossed with a dwarf, pear fruited plant. The cross produced 91 tall spherical, 119 dwarf pear, 38 tall pear and 52 dwarf spherical. Another tall plant with spherical fruit (Cross-II) was crossed with dwarf, pear-fruited plant and the progeny produced were tall pear 23, dwarf spherical 19, tall spherical 7 and dwarf pear 11. Present the results diagrammatically showing the genetic markers on the chromosomes. If the two tall plants with spherical fruit were crossed with each other, i.e. I × II, what phenotypic classes are expected from this cross and in what proportions?

5.2 CHROMOSOME ABNORMALITIES

The genetic diseases can occur at two levels: genic and chromosomes. Some of the abnormalities occurring at gene level (genic mutations) and gross chromosomes in humans are:

S. no.	Abnormality/disease	Major symptoms
	(a) Chromosome Abnormalities	
1	Klinefelter's Syndrome	XXY sex chromosomes (44+XXY; 44+XXXY), sterile males, may show some female features; Feminine pitched voice, long limbs and knock knees
2	XYY Syndrome	Extra Y in males; individuals exhibit normal development and above average height, tendency to delayed mental maturation with an increased probability for learning problems
3	Metafemales – XXX	Extra X in females (44+XXX); normal development and sexual characteristics, usually taller than other females with some learning difficulties
4	Down's Syndrome (Trisomy 21)	Extra chromosome 21 results in mental retardation, heart defects, more likely to occur in infants born to older women
5	Turner's Syndrome (X_)	Females lack one X-chromosome, some mental retardation, results in sterility, short in stature, never develop ovaries, increased incidence of thyroid problems.
6	Non-disjunction during Meiosis	Some gametes contain extra chromosome, other gametes are missing chromosome
7	Cri du Chat Syndrome	Broken chromosome, results in retardation, malformed larynx and vocal problems
8	Fragile X-Syndrome	Broken chromosome, results in sterility, mental retardation, oversized testes in males, double jointedness
	(b) Genic Abnormalities	
1	Hemophilia	Homozygous recessive, blood-clotting problem, victims bleeds to death

2	Sickle-cell anemia	Lack proper blood protein and RBCs are sickle shaped, unable to carry oxygen efficiency; due to recessive allele, causes a simple substitution
3	Phenylketonuria	Unable to produce enzymes to breakdown chemicals in diet soda can lead to toxic buildup and death; due to recessive allele
4	Galactosemia	Unable to produce enzymes necessary for breakdown of galactose in milk, toxic buildup; due to recessive allele. Galactosemia is not lactose intolerance, which is not a genetic disease, occurs over time with aging
5	Lesch-Nyhan disease	Missing an enzyme necessary for purine metabolism, leading to hyperpuricemia, severe mental retardation, self-mutilation and renal failure; X-linked recessive disease
6	Huntington's Disease	Deterioration of nervous system; due to dominant allele
7	Achondroplastic dwarfism	Small stature, disproportionate limbs, short broad hands and feet, waddling gait; due to dominant allele; affects bone growth beginning at birth; usually does not affect intelligence but psychological problems may occur when child realizes he/she is different

HOME WORK

5.2.1 The Drosophila fourth chromosome is so small that flies monosomic or trisomic for it survive and are fertile. Several genes, including *eyeless* (*ey*), have been located on this chromosome. If a cytologically normal fly homozygous for a recessive eyeless mutation is crossed to a fly monosomic for a wild-type fourth chromosome, what kinds of progeny will be produced and in what proportions?

5.2.2 In cattle, the normal diploid chromosome number (2n) is 60. What is the chromosome content in the following:

(a) a monosomic   (b) a double monosomic

(c) a tetrasomic   (d) a double trisomic

(e) a tetraploid   (f) a hexaploid

5.2.3   A plant species has 14 chromosomes while the another had tetraploid 28 chromosomes. Hybrids between these two species are sterile F_1 individuals. Some unreduced gametes of the F_1 are functional in backcrosses. Find out the chromosome number and level of *ploidy* for each of the following:

(a) F_1; (b) F_1 backcrossed to parent with 14 chromosomes; (c) F_1 backcrossed to parent with 28 chromosomes; (d) Chromosome doubling of F_1.

5.2.4   (a) How will you synthesize a pentaploid (5n)?

(b) How do you synthesize a triploid and tetraploid genotypes Aaa and Aaaa?

5.2.5   The diploid chromosome number in garden peas is 14. (a) How many different trisomics could be formed? (b) How many different double trisomics could be formed?

5.2.6   A woman with X-linked colour blindness and Turner syndrome had a colour blind father and a normal mother. In which of her parents did nondisjunction of the sex chromosomes occur?

5.2.7   In cattle, eight regions of chromosome were detected, out of which four are given below. Assuming that the new races were evolved by single inversion from the earlier sequences, show how the four races could have been originated.

(a) Ahbdcfeg   (b) aedcfbhg   (c) ahbdgefc   (d) aefcdbhg

5.2.8   If the gene sequence on one of the autosomes is A B C D E F and on another is M N O P Q R and a reciprocal translocation between these two chromosomes produced the two chromosomes with the gene order: A B C P Q R on one chromosome and M N O D E F on the other, illustrate how these translocated chromosomes would pair with their normal counterparts in a heterozygous individual during Meiosis?

5.2.9   A yellow-bodied Drosophila female with attached X-chromosome was crossed to a white-eyed male. Both of the parental phenotypes are caused by X-linked recessive mutations. Predict the phenotypes of the progeny.

5.2.10 In Drosophila, the autosomal genes *cinnabar* (*cn*) and *brown* (*bw*) control the production of brown and red eye pigments, respectively. Flies homozygous for *cinnabar* mutations have bright red eyes, flies homozygous for *brown* mutations have brown eyes, and flies homozygous for mutations in both of these genes have white eyes. A male homozygous for mutations in the *cn* and *bw* genes has bright red eyes because a small duplication that carries the wild-type allele of *bw* (*bw*+) is attached to the Y-chromosome. If this male is mated to a karyotypically normal female that is homozygous for the *cn* and *bw* mutations, what types of progeny will be produced?

5.2.11 The genes for vermilion (*v*) eyes, sable (*s*) body colour and forked bristles (*f*) are on the X-chromosome of *Drosophila melanogaster*. They map in the order *v s f*, with 10 map units between *v* and *s* and 14 map units between *s* and *f*. Suppose that you cross a wild-type male with a *v s f* female and then test cross the F_1 females.

(a) Indicate the progeny classes and their expected numbers among 2000 total progeny, assuming that interference, i = 1.

(b) Make the same calculation assuming an interference value of i = 0.5

(c) Assume again that I = 1 and suppose that you cross a homozygous wild-type female to a v s f male and then mate the progeny among themselves. What are the possible classes of progeny and their expected numbers among 2000 progeny animals?

5.2.12 The gel diagram given below shows the banding pattern corresponding to restriction-fragment length polymorphism (RFLPs) in each of two genes, one with alleles called A and a and the other with alleles called B and b. The banding patterns of the parents P_1 and P_2 are shown on the left of the diagram. The number of each possible type of banding pattern observed among 200 offsprings is shown at the right. (a) What is the genotype of the parent P_1? (b) What is the frequency of recombination of between A and B?

	Parents			Offspring			
	P_1	P_2		22	85	75	18
A	– – – – – – – – – – – – –			– – – – – – – – – – – – –	– – – – – – – – – – – – –		
a	– – – – – – – – – – – – –	– – – – – – – – – – – – –		– – – – – – – – – – – – –	– – – – – – – – – – – – –	– – – – – – – – – – – – –	– – – – – – – – – – – – –
B	– – – – – – – – – – – – –			– – – – – – – – – – – – –		– – – – – – – – – – – – –	
b	– – – – – – – – – – – – –	– – – – – – – – – – – – –		– – – – – – – – – – – – –	– – – – – – – – – – – – –	– – – – – – – – – – – – –	– – – – – – – – – – – – –

PRACTICAL NO. 6

6.1 CALCULATION OF GENE FREQUENCY WHEN THE DOMINANCE IS INCOMPLETE

For the traits, where there is no dominance or dominance is lacking, the genotypes of the individuals in a population may be determined from their phenotypes. The estimation of gene frequency under such condition is outlined below, with the help of an example.

CLASS WORK

1. The coat colour in mice is determined by two alleles C and c. The genotypes CC, Cc and cc produce yellow, cream and white colours, respectively. In a sample of 600 mice under random mating, 150 were yellow, 250 cream and 200 white. Calculate the genotype frequencies and gene frequency of yellow and white genes and test whether the population is under Hardy-Weinberg equilibrium.

    (a) Calculation of genotype frequency:

Phenotype	Genotype	No. of animals	Genotype frequency
Yellow	CC	150	$150 \div 600 = 0.25$
Cream	Cc	250	$250 \div 600 = 0.42$
White	Cc	200	$200 \div 600 = 0.33$

    (b) Calculation of gene frequency:

    (i) The gene frequency may be obtained from the genotype frequencies as:

Phenotype	Genotype	No. of animals	No. of genes		
			C	c	Total
Yellow	CC	150	300	0	300
Cream	Cc	250	250	250	500
White	cc	200	0	400	400
	Total	600	550	650	1200

Gene frequency of yellow gene (p) = 550 ÷ 1200 = 0.46

Gene frequency of white gene (q) = 650 ÷ 1200 = 0.54

Check: p + q will be always sum to unity, i.e. 0.46 + 0.54 = 1.00.

(ii) Calculation of gene frequency from genotype frequency:

The genotype frequencies observed are:

CC (D) = 0.25; Cc (H) = 0.42; and cc (R) = 0.33

Frequency of yellow gene (p)	=	D + ½ H
	=	0.25 + ½ (0.42)
	=	0.46
Frequency of white gene (q)	=	R + ½ H
	=	0.33 + ½ (0.42)
	=	0.54

(c) Test for the Hardy-Weinberg equilibrium by using chi-square test of significance

The chi-square test is applied to compare the observed and expected frequencies. It measures the departure of the observed frequencies (O) from the expected frequencies (E), and it is calculated as the sum of the ratios of the squared deviations of the observed from the expected frequencies to the expected frequency.

The chi-square is computed as:

$$\chi^2 = \sum \frac{(O - E)^2}{R}$$

The null hypothesis (H_0) for the chi-square test assumes that there is no significant difference between the observed and expected frequencies. The expected genotype frequencies with the gene frequencies p = 0.46 and q = 0.54 are:

$(0.46 + 0.54)^2 = (0.46)^2 + 2 (0.46 \times 0.54) + (0.54)^2$

$\qquad\qquad = 0.21 + 0.50 + 0.29$

The expected number of animals of different phenotypes is

Yellow = 0.21 × 600 = 126

Cream = 0.50 × 600 = 300

White = 0.29 × 600 = 174

Genotype	Observed no. (O)	Expected no. (E)	(O − E)	(O − E)^2	(O − E)^2/E
CC	150	126	24	576	4.57
Cc	250	300	-50	2500	8.33
cc	200	174	26	676	3.89
Total	600	600			16.79

The chi-square calculated value is compared with the chi-square table value at (k − r) degrees of freedom, where k is the number of phenotypes and r is the number of alleles. In the present case, it is 3 − 2 = 1 d.f. The chi-square table value at 1 d.f. with 5% level of significance is 3.84.

Conclusion: Since the chi-square calculated value (16.79) is more than the tabulated value (3.84), the null hypothesis is rejected; and it is concluded that there is a significant difference between the observed and expected frequencies. In other words, the population is not under Hardy-Weinberg equilibrium.

Chi-square table values:

d.f.	5% L.S.	1% L.S.
1	3.84	6.63
2	5.99	9.21
3	7.81	11.34

2. Coat colour in Shorthorn cattle is influenced by a pair of codominant alleles 'R' for Red and 'r' for white. In a herd of 1000 Shorthorn cattle, there were 600 red (RR), 300 roan (Rr) and remaining white. Calculate the genotype frequencies of red, roan and white genotypes and gene frequencies of red and white genes. Also test whether the population is under Hardy-Weinberg equilibrium.

The genotypic frequencies can be calculated as follows:

Phenotype	Genotype	No. of animals	Genotypic frequency
Red	RR	600	600/1000 = 0.60 or 60%
Roan	Rr	300	300/1000 = 0.30 or 30%
White	Rr	100	100/1000 = 0.10 or 10%
Total		1000	1.00 or 100%

Gene frequencies can be calculated by any one of the following three methods.

(a) Gene counting method:

Phenotype	Genotype	No. of animals	Number of alleles		
			Red (R)	White (r)	Total
Red	RR	600	1200	0	1200
Roan	Rr	300	300	300	600
White	Rr	100	0	200	200
Total		1000	1500	500	2000

Frequency of red allele = Number of red alleles ÷ Total number of alleles
= 1500 ÷ 2000 = 0.75 or 75%
Frequency of white allele = Number of white alleles ÷ Total number of alleles
= 500 ÷ 2000 = 0.25 or 25%

(b) From the number of genotypes:

$$\text{Frequency of red allele } (C^R) = p = \frac{D + \frac{1}{2}H}{N}, \text{ where}$$

D = Number of dominant genotypes = 60
H = Number of heterozygous genotypes = 30
N = Total number of genotypes = 100

$$p = \frac{60 + \frac{1}{2}(30)}{100} = \frac{75}{100} = 0.75 \text{ or } 75\%$$

$$\text{Frequency of white allele } (C^w) = q = \frac{R = \frac{1}{2}H}{N} = \frac{25}{100} = 0.25 \text{ or } 25\% =$$

Alternately, gene frequencies can also be estimated from the genotype frequencies as:
Frequency of $C^R = p = p^2 + \frac{1}{2}(2 pq) = 0.60 + \frac{1}{2}(0.30) = 0.60 + 0.15 = 0.75$
Frequency of $C^r = q = q^2 + \frac{1}{2}(2 pq) = 0.10 + \frac{1}{2}(0.30) = 0.10 + 0.15 = 0.25$

(c) Testing for Hardy-Weinberg equilibrium:
Testing for Hardy-Weinberg equilibrium means testing whether the genotypic frequencies observed in the population are in accordance with the frequencies predicted by the Hardy-Weinberg equilibrium.
If the two alleles, say p and q, are allele frequencies in Hardy-Weinberg equilibrium, the frequencies of the homozygous dominants, heterozygotes and homozygous recessives expected would be p^2, 2pq and q^2, respectively. The statistical significance between the observed and expected frequencies can be tested by Chi-square test. The null

hypothesis (H_0) formulated will be that the number of animals of different genotypes in the population are in accordance with those expected under Hardy-Weinberg equilibrium.

Phenotype	Genotype	Observed frequency (O)	Expected frequency (E)	(O − E)	(O − E)²/E
Red	$C^R C^R$	600	$1000 \times 0.75^2 = 562.50$	37.5	2.5
Roan	$C^R C^r$	300	$1000 \times 2 \times 0.75 \times$ $0.25 = 375$	−75.0	15.0
White	$C^r C^r$	100	$1000 \times 0.25^2 = 62.50$	37.5	22.5
Total		1000			40.0

Chi-square table value at (k − r) d.f., where k is the number of phenotypic classes and r is the number of alleles involved, i.e. 3 − 2 = 1, d.f. = 3.84 and 6.63 at 5% and 1% level of significance, respectively. Since the Chi-square calculated value is higher than the table value at 1% LS, the null hypothesis formulated is rejected (P < 0.01), and it is concluded that there is a highly significant difference between the observed and expected frequencies. In other words, the population is not under Hardy-Weinberg equilibrium.

HOME WORK

6.1.1   In a certain plant, the cross purple × blue yields purple- and blue-flowered progeny in equal proportions, but blue × blue always gives rise only to blue. (a) What does this tell you about the genotypes of blue- and purple-flowered plants? (b) Which phenotype is dominant?

6.1.2   The inheritance of different types of earwax was studied among the people. It was observed that an individual could have one of the two types of earwax, dry or sticky, which were inherited in the fashion shown by the following data:

Parental combination	Number of matings	Offspring	
		Sticky	Dry
Sticky × sticky	9	30	6
Sticky × dry	9	21	10
Dry × dry	13	0	44

On the basis of these data, explain whether the inheritance of dry earwax is caused by dominance, recessiveness, partial dominance, codominance or some other mode.

6.1.3 In Shorthorn cattle, the heterozygous condition of the alleles for red coat colour (R) and white coat colour (r). (a) If two roan cattle are mated, what proportion of the progeny will resemble their parents in coat colour? (b) What progeny will a roan Shorthorn have if bred to: (i) red, (ii) roan and (iii) white?

6.1.4 In four o'clock plants, the allele for red flower colour has an effect that is incompletely dominant over the effect of the white colour allele. If a cross between two plants produced 18 red, 32 pink and 15 white plants, what are the phenotypes of the parents?

6.1.5 A plant population consists of two types of flowers – white and red, controlled by a single locus and two alleles. The white represents the recessive homozygote, while the red consists of some combination of heterozygotes and dominant homozygotes. Assume that 50% of the population has red flowers. What are the frequencies of all three genotypes assuming Hardy-Weinberg equilibrium?

6.1.6 Which of the following genotype frequencies of AA, Aa and aa, respectively, satisfy the Hardy-Weinberg law?

(a) 0.25, 0.50, 0.25 (b) 0.36, 0.55, 0.09 (c) 0.49, 0.42, 0.09
(d) 0.64, 0.27, 0.09 (e) 0.29, 0.42, 0.29

6.1.7 A population geneticist observed the RFLP phenotypes given in following diagram, where the number above each well is the number of individuals exhibiting the corresponding phenotype. Test whether the observed phenotype frequencies are consistent with those expected from a single locus with three alleles in a random-mating population, using the chi-square test. Explain why the appropriate number of degrees of freedom in this test is 3.

No. of individuals					
18	68	90	115	360	349
-----------	------------		------------		
	------------	------------		------------	
			------------	------------	-----------

6.2 CALCULATION OF GENE FREQUENCY WHEN THE DOMINANCE IS COMPLETE

For the traits where the dominance is complete, the genotypes cannot be determined from the phenotypes because the homozygous dominant and heterozygous genotypes are indistinguishable phenotypically. For such traits, the gene frequency may be determined by using the Hardy-Weinberg law, from the equation q = square root of q^2, where q^2 is the genotype frequency of homozygous recessive genotype.

CLASS WORK

1. In cattle, the black coat colour (B) is completely dominant over the red (b). In a sample of 450 animals under random mating, 72 were red. Calculate the gene frequency of black and red genes and find out the number of heterozygous carriers.

   Frequency of red genotype = 72/450 = 0.16

   Frequency of red gene (q) = square root of 0.16 = 0.4

   Therefore, the frequency of black gene (p) = (1 – 0.40 = 0.60)

   The proportion of heterozygous animals = 2pq = 2 × 0.6 × 0.4 = 0.48

   Number of heterozygous carriers = 450 × 0.48 = 216

2. In humans, the red-green colour blindness is due to a sex-linked recessive gene (c). In a random mating population, about 8% of the men were colour blind. Assuming the population to be under Hardy-Weinberg equilibrium, (a) what percentage of women would be expected to be colour blind? (b) What percentage of the women is expected to be heterozygous? (c) What percentage of men would be expected to have normal vision after two generations?

   Since the colour blindness is sex-linked recessive in males, the single gene on X chromosome is sufficient for its expression. Therefore, in males, the gene frequency of recessive gene is equal to the genotype frequency of recessive genotype. Let q be the frequency of recessive genotype (cc) = gene frequency = q = 8/100 = 0.08.

   Therefore, the frequency of dominant gene, p = (1 – q) = (1 – 0.08) = 0.92.

   (a) Frequency of colour-blind women is q^2 = $(0.08)^2$ = 0.0064 or 0.64%, i.e. 0.64% of the women in the given population are expected to be colour blind.

(b) Frequency of heterozygous women is given by $2pq = 2 \times 0.08 \times 0.92 = 0.1472$ or 14.72 percent of the population are expected to be heterozygous carriers.

(c) In a population under random mating and Hardy-Weinberg equilibrium, the gene frequencies and genotype frequencies will not change from generation to generation. Therefore, the genotype frequency of normal men after two generations would be expected to remain same as 0.92 or 92%.

HOME WORK

6.2.1 Coat colour in dairy cattle is governed by two alleles. The allele B for black colour is completely dominant over the allele for red colour b. The frequency of red animals in the same flock was found to be 16%.

(a) Calculate the frequency of black (B) and red (b) alleles.

(b) Calculate the expected frequencies of three genotypes.

(c) What percentage of all the black animals is expected to be carriers of b allele?

6.2.2 A population has been maintained by mating randomly for many generations and two phenotypes are segregating. One is due to the dominant allele G and the other to a recessive allele g. The frequencies of the dominant and recessive phenotypes were 0.7975 and 0.2025, respectively. Estimate the frequencies of dominant and recessive alleles.

(a) Calculate the frequency of heterozygotes Aa in a randomly mating population if the frequency of recessive phenotypes is 0.08.

(b) The incidence of recessive albinism in a human population is 0.008. If the mating for this trait is random in this population, calculate the frequency of recessive allele.

(c) The frequency of an allele in a large randomly mating population was 0.80. What is the frequency of heterozygous carriers?

(d) In human beings, the gene for taster (T) to the substance phenylthiocarbamide (PTC) is dominant to non-taster. (i) Calculate the gene frequencies of T and t if there were 78 tasters out of 100 persons tested in a population. (ii) If the frequency of T allele in a population is 0.4, what is the probability that a particular taster is homozygous?

6.2.3   In mice, the black coat colour (B) is dependent upon a dominant allele and the brown colour on its recessive allele (b). If a random sample of 800 mice has 738 black and 62 brown animals, calculate the frequencies of black and brown genes.

6.2.4   In a large random mating population, 84% of the individuals express the dominant phenotype of an allele A (AA) and 16% express the phenotype of the recessive allele a (aa). (a) What is the frequency of dominant allele? (b) If aa homozygotes are 5% less fit than the other two genotypes, what will be the frequency of A in the next generation?

6.2.5   The frequency of infants homozygous for recessive abnormality in a population was about 1 in 25,000. What is the expected frequency of heterozygous carriers in the population?

6.2.6   Albinism is due to recessive genotype (aa). If one out of every 18,000 individuals in a population was an albino, what percentage of the population is heterozygous for this gene?

6.2.7   The genotype frequencies of three genotypes AA, Aa and aa, in two populations under Hardy-Weinberg equilibrium are given below.

Genotype:	AA	Aa	aa
Frequency in population I	0.04	0.32	0.64
Frequency in population II	0.64	0.32	0.04

(a) If the populations are equal in size and they merge to form a single large population, predict the allele and genotype frequencies in the large population immediately after merger.

(b) If the merged population reproduces by random mating, predict the genotype frequencies in the next generation.

(c) If the merged population continues to reproduce by random mating, will these genotype frequencies remain constant?

6.2.8   The wire-haired texture (W) in dogs is dominant over the smooth-haired one (w). A random mating population of 500 dogs was found to contain 75% wire-haired individuals. In such a case (a) calculate the frequencies of dominant and recessive alleles and frequencies of dominant homozygous, recessive homozygous and carriers of recessive allele for smooth hair; and (b) If the parental population mates at random and produces 100 offspring, calculate the expected number of individuals belonging to each genotype.

6.2.9   Consider the gene for Rh factor. Let R be the allele for Rh$^+$ and r be the allele for Rh$^-$, such that RR and Rr are Rh$^+$ and rr is Rh$^-$. Assume a large population in equilibrium in which 16% of the individuals are Rh$^-$.

(a) What is the calculated frequency of the r allele? Of the R allele?

(b) What is the calculated frequency of the genotypes in this population?

(c) An Rh$^+$ man marries an Rh$^-$ woman. What is the probability that the man is heterozygous (Rr)? That he is homozygous (RR)? What is the probability that this couple's first child will be Rh$^-$?

6.2.10   A random mating population of dairy cattle contains an autosomal recessive allele causing dwarfism. In a herd, if the frequency of dwarf calves is 10 percent, what is the frequency of heterozygous carriers of the allele in the entire herd? What is the frequency of heterozygotes among the non-dwarf cattle?

6.2.11   In a population, if the frequencies of alleles determining the A, B, O blood groups were estimated as 0.10, 0.74 and 0.16, respectively. Assuming random mating, what are the expected frequencies of ABO genotypes and phenotypes?

6.2.12   If an X-linked recessive trait is present in 2 percent of the males in a population with random mating, what is the frequency of the trait in females? What is the frequency of carrier females?

6.2.13   Among the 35 flowering plant population, the following genotypes were observed of the enzyme *phosphoglucose isomerase* as: 2 A_1A_1, 13 A_1A_2, 20 A_2A_2. (a) What are the frequencies of alleles A_1 and A_2? (b) Assuming random mating, what is the expected number of genotypes?

6.2.14   Xenoderma pigmentosa (XP) is a fatal skin cancer, resulting from a recessive mutant allele that affects the DNA repair. If the frequency of homozygous recessive affected individuals is approximately one in 2,50,000, (a) what is the expected frequency of XP among the offspring of first-cousin matings? (b) What is the ratio of XP among the offspring of first-cousin matings to that among the offspring of non-relatives?

6.2.15 Sickle cell anemia is a genetic disease in human beings. The homozygous-dominant individuals (SS) are normal but easily infected with malarial parasite, become ill and may die, whereas the individuals homozygous for sickle cell trait (ss) have the red blood cells, which easily collapse under low oxygen condition. The malarial parasite cannot grow in these cells but the individuals die due to genetic defect. The heterozygous individuals (Ss), however, have some sick red blood cells, partially defective. Malarial parasite cannot survive in these partially defective cells. Thus, heterozygous individuals can survive better than either of the homozygous individuals. In a population, if 9% of the individuals are suffering from sickle cell anemia, what percentage of this population are resistant to malaria because of the heterozygous (Ss) genotype.

6.2.16 The percentage of homozygous recessive genotype (aa) in a population is 36%. Based on this, calculate the frequencies of 'aa' genotype, 'a' allele, 'A' allele and genotypes 'AA' and 'Aa'.

6.2.17 In mice, white coloring is caused by the double recessive genotype 'aa'. In a large random mating population, 35% were white. Calculate the allelic and genotypic frequencies for this population.

6.2.18 In a population of butterflies, the color brown (B) is dominant over the color white (b) and 40% of all butterflies are white. With this simple information, calculate the percentage of butterflies in the population that are heterozygous and frequency of homozygous-dominant individuals.

6.3 CALCULATION OF GENE FREQUENCY FOR MULTIPLE ALLELES

Three or more genes, any one of which may occupy same locus in homologous chromosome pair is called multiple alleles. Assume that in a population under random mating, the gene frequency of three alleles influencing a trait to be p, q and r, then the genotype frequencies are distributed as:

$$(p + q + r)^2 = p^2 + 2pq + 2pr + q^2 + 2qr + r^2$$

Sum of the gene frequencies as well as the genotype frequencies is always unity.

CLASS WORK

(a) When the Dominance Is Hierarchical Among the Multiple Alleles

Coat colour in rabbits is governed by the multiple alleles. The full colour (C), Himalayan (c^h) and albino (c) form a multiple allelic series, with the dominance in that order. In a population under random mating, there were 672 full coloured, 120 Himalayan and 8 albino rabbits. Find out the gene frequencies of full colour, Himalayan and albino genes.

$(p + q + r)^2 = p^2 + 2pq + 2pr + q^2 + 2qr + r^2$, where

$p^2 + 2pq + 2pr$ = genotype frequency of full colour with Cc, Cc^h and Cc genotypes

$q^2 + 2qr$ = genotype frequency of Himalayan with c^hc^h and

r^2 = genotype frequency of albino with cc genotype

The observed frequencies are:

Full colour = 672/800 = 0.84

Himalayan = 120/800 = 0.15

Albino = 8/800 = 0.01

    (i)   Gene frequency of albino (c) = r = square root of 0.01 = 0.1 since gene frequency is equal to square root of genotype frequency.

   (ii)   Genotype frequency of Himalayan (c^h) = $q^2 + 2qr$

           But $(q + r)^2 = q^2 + 2qr + r^2$

           Therefore, $(q + r)$ = square root of $(q^2 + 2qr + r^2)$

           Hence, q = square root of $(q^2 + 2qr + r^2) - r$

$(q^2 + 2qr)$ = genotype frequency of Himalayan = 0.15

r^2 = genotype frequency of albino = 0.01

r = gene frequency of albino gene = 0.1

Now, substitute these values in the above equation,

q = [square root of (0.15 + 0.01)] – 0.1 = 0.4 – 0.1 = 0.32

(ii) Gene frequency of full colour (C) = p = (1 – p – r) since p + q + r = 1

r = 0.1, q = 0.3, therefore p = (1 – 0.3 – 0.1) = 0.6

(b) When Codominance Is Involved in Multiple Alleles

In man, the A, B, O blood groups are governed by the multiple allelic series with codominance among these alleles involved. In a population under Hardy-Weinberg equilibrium, 42, 8, 3 and 47 per cent belong to A, B, AB and O blood groups, respectively. Find out the gene frequencies of A, B and O genes. Also find out the estimated phenotype frequencies of the four blood groups in a sample of 500 people.

Let p, q and r be the gene frequencies of I^A, I^B and i alleles, respectively. The phenotypes, possible genotypes, the observed and expected genotype frequencies among the offspring are as follows:

Blood group	Possible genotypes	Genotype frequency	
		Observed	Expected
A	$I^A I^A$, $I^A i$	0.42	$p^2 + 2pr$
B	$I^B I^B$, $I^B i$	0.42	$q^2 + 2qr$
O	Ii	0.47	r^2
AB	$I^A I^B$	0.03	2pq

(i) Gene frequency of allele i = r = square root of r^2 = square root of 0.47 = 0.69

(ii) Gene frequency of allele I^A = p = $(p + r)^2$ = $p^2 + 2pr + r^2$

Therefore, (p + r) = square root of $(p^2 + 2pr + r^2)$

Hence, p = square root of $(p^2 + 2pr + r^2)$ – r

By substituting the values of

$p^2 + 2pr$ = 0.42; r^2 = 0.47 and r = 0.69 in the last equation,

p = square root of (0.42 + 0.47) – 0.69

= 0.94 – 0.69 = 0.25

(iii) Gene frequency of allele IB = q = (1 – p – r) = (1 – 0.25 – 0.69) = 0.06

(iv) The estimated phenotype frequencies of different blood groups in a sample of 500 people are:

Blood group A   =   N $\{p^2 + 2pr\}$, where N = 500

                  =   500 $\{(0.25)^2 + 2(0.25)\,(0.69)\}$

                  = $500 \times 0.4075 = 204$

Blood group B   =   N $\{q^2 + 2qr\}$, where N = 500

                  =   500 $\{(0.06)^2 + 2(0.06)\,(0.69)\}$

                  = $500 \times 0.0864 = 43$

Blood group O   =   N $\{r^2\}$, where N = 500

                  =   500 $\{(0.69)^2\}$

                  = $500 \times 0.4761 = 238$

Blood group AB =   N $\{2pq\}$, where N = 500

                  =   500 $\{2 \times 0.25 \times 0.06\}$

                  = $500 \times 0.03 = 15$

6.4 TESTING THE MENDELIAN SEGREGATION RATIOS AND HARDY-WEINBERG EQUILIBRIUM

In a large random mating population, the genotype frequencies and gene frequencies remain unaltered from generation to generation in the absence of migration, mutation and selection and the genotype frequencies can be determined from the gene frequencies.

The formulae of Hardy-Weinberg allow us to determine whether evolution has occurred. Any changes in the gene frequencies in the population over time can be detected. The law states that if no evolution is occurring, then an equilibrium of allele frequencies will remain in effect in each succeeding generation of sexually reproducing individuals. If the equilibrium to remain in effect (i.e. that no evolution is occurring), then the following five conditions must be met:

- The population must be large enough so that no genetic drift (random chance) can cause the allele frequencies to change.
- Random mating must occur, i.e. individuals must pair by chance.
- No mutations must occur so that new alleles do not enter the population.
- No gene flow can occur, i.e. no migration of individuals into, or out of the population.
- No selection can occur so that certain alleles are not selected for, or against.

Obviously, the Hardy-Weinberg equilibrium cannot exist in real life. Some or all of these types of forces act on living populations at various times, and evolution at some level occurs in all living organisms. The Hardy-Weinberg formulae allow us to detect some allele frequencies that change from generation to generation, thus allowing a simplified method of determining that evolution is occurring. There are two formulas that must be memorized:

$p^2 + 2pq + q^2 = 1$ and $p + q = 1$, where

p = frequency of the dominant allele in the population

q = frequency of the recessive allele in the population

p^2 = percentage of homozygous-dominant individuals

q^2 = percentage of homozygous-recessive individuals

$2pq$ = percentage of heterozygous individuals

Gene frequency: Gene frequency is defined as the proportion or frequency of a gene in relation to its allele at a locus in the population. It refers to the relative abundance or relative rarity of a particular gene in population, as compared to its own allele in that population. The frequency of a gene varies from zero to one. For example, if A1 is an allele at the locus A, the gene frequency of A1 gene is proportion or percentage of all genes at this locus that are the A1 alleles.

The gene frequency at a locus among a group of individuals can be determined from the genotype frequencies. Suppose there are 2 alleles, A_1 and A_2, at a locus A, then the relationship between gene and genotype frequencies is as follows:

	Genes		Genotypes		
	A_1	A_2	A_1A_1	A_1A_2	A_2A_2
Frequencies	p	q	D	H	R

The genotype frequencies of A_1A_1, A_1A_2 and A_2A_2 genotypes will be $D \div N$, $H \div N$ and $R \div N$, respectively, where N is the total number of individuals in the population. Then, the gene frequency of A_1 gene is $p = D + \frac{1}{2} H$ and the gene frequency of A_2 gene is $q = R + \frac{1}{2} H$. In a population, $p + q = 1$ and similarly, $D + H + R = 1$.

CLASS WORK

1. Mendel test crossed pea plants grown from yellow (seed colour), round (seed shape) F_1 seeds to plants grown from green, wrinkled seeds and obtained the following results: 30 yellow, round; 28 yellow, wrinkled; 35 green, round; and 27 green, wrinkled. Are these results consistent with the hypothesis that seed colour and seed shape are controlled by independently assorting genes, each segregating two alleles?

Phenotype	Genotype	Observed number	Expected frequency	Expected number	Obs. no. − Exp. no.	(Obs. No. − Exp. no.)²/Exp.
Yellow, round	Y_R_	30	9/16 = 0.5625	120 × 0.5625 = 67.5	(30 − 67.5) = −37.5	20.83
Yellow, wrinkled	Y_rr	28	3/16 = 0.1875	120 × 0.175 = 22.5	(28 − 22.5) = 5.5	1.34

Green, round	yyR_	35	3/16 = 0.1875	120 × 0.175 = 22.5	(35 – 22.5) = 12.5	6.94
Green, wrinkled	yyrr	27	1/16 = 0.0625	120 × 0.0625 = 7.50	(27 – 7.5) = 19.5	50.70
Total		120	1.0000	120		79.81

First, the null hypothesis is formulated that the genes responsible for seed colour segregate independent of the seed shape or the number of plants obtained are in accordance with the Mendel's dihybrid inheritance. The expected frequencies of the four classes under dihybrid inheritance are calculated. For example, the expected frequency of yellow, round is 9 out of 16, which comes to a ratio of 0.5625. Similarly, the expected frequencies of yellow, wrinkled; green, round; and green wrinkled classes, calculated in the same manner are 0.1875, 0.1875 and 0.0625, respectively. Then, for each of the four classes, the expected numbers are obtained by multiplying the expected frequency with total number of plants, i.e. 120. In the next step, the difference between observed and expected numbers are estimated, and the difference for each class is squared and divided by the expected number of individuals for each of the four classes. The values obtained for four classes are summed to get the total chi-square calculated value (79.81), which is compared with the chi-square table value at $(k - 1)$ d.f., at 5% or 1% level of significance, where k is the number of classes tested. The chi-square table values at 2 d.f. are 5.991 and 9.210 at 5% and 1% level of significance, respectively. If the chi-square calculated value is equal to or less than the table value, null hypothesis is accepted otherwise rejected and concluded accordingly. In the present case, since the chi-square calculated value is more than the table value even at 1% level of significance, we reject the null hypothesis and conclude that the genes responsible for seed colour and seed shape did not segregate independently. The parental combination of yellow, round seeds is much less (30) than the expected numbers (67.5).

2. The number of genotypes of AA, Aa and aa in a sample of 134 animals in a village were 68, 42 and 24, respectively. Calculate the frequencies of A and a alleles. Predict the Hardy-Weinberg genotype frequencies with the help of allele frequencies obtained and test whether the observed frequencies are in agreement with the expected frequencies.

Frequency of A allele, $p = [(2 \times 68) + 42] / (2 \times 134) = 0.66$

Frequency of a allele, $q = [(2 \times 24) + 42] / (2 \times 134) = 0.34$

We formulate the null hypothesis that the observed frequencies are in agreement with the expected frequencies.

The agreement of observed frequencies with the expected ones can be tested by chi-square test as shown below.

Genotype	Observed number	Expected frequency	Expected number	Obs. – Exp. No.	(Obs. – Exp. No.)^2/ Exp.
AA	68	$p^2 = 0.44$	59.0	9.0	1.37
Aa	42	$2pq = 0.45$	60.3	−18.3	5.55
Aa	24	$q^2 = 0.11$	14.7	9.3	5.88
Total	134	1.000	134.0		12.80

The calculated chi-square value (12.80) exceeds the critical values of 5.991 and 9.210 at 2 d.f., 5% and 1% level of significance, respectively. Hence, we reject the hypothesis that the genotype frequencies calculated from the Hardy-Weinberg principle agree with observed frequencies. Evidently, the population is not in Hardy-Weinberg equilibrium.

HOME WORK

6.4.1   Conduct a chi-square test to determine if an observed ratio of 30 tall: 20 dwarf pea plants is consistent with the expected ratio of 1:1 from the cross Tt × tt?

6.4.2   Mendel crossed pea plants producing round seeds with those producing wrinkled seeds. From a total of 7324 F_2 seeds, 5474 were round and 1850 were wrinkled. Using the symbols W and w for genes, (a) symbolize the original P cross, (b) the gametes and (c) F_1 progeny; (d) represent a cross between two F_1 plants (or one selfed); (e) symbolize the gametes; and (f) summarize the expected F_2 results under the headings: phenotypes, genotypes, genotypic frequency and phenotypic ratio.

6.4.3   A population is in Hardy-Weinberg equilibrium. Consider only a single locus and two alleles found at that locus. If the frequency of a allele is 0.4, what is the frequency of all of the possible genotypes at this locus. Call the other allele A.

6.4.4   A population consists of 200 aa individuals and is in Hardy-Weinberg equilibrium. Assuming one-locus, two allele genetics, what is the frequency of *a* allele if the population consists of a total of 1000 individuals? What if the 200 *aa* individual population consists of a total of 10,000 individuals?

6.4.5   A population is in Hardy-Weinberg equilibrium. The frequency of the dominant phenotype is 0.99. What fraction of individuals that carry at least one recessive allele are homozygous at this locus?

6.4.6   In a hypothetical population of 2500 people, 2275 have brown eyes and 225 have blue eyes (the homozygous recessive phenotype). If there are 4000 children produced by this generation, how many of the children would be expected to be heterozygous for the eye colour?

6.4.7   In a human population, if the gene B is responsible for brown eyes and b is for blue eyes and given a population consisting of 323 BB, 23 Bb and 45 bb, what are the frequencies of allele B and of allele b? Is the population under Hardy-Weinberg equilibrium? Quantitatively justify your answer.

6.4.8   Suppose a population has started with 20% blue-eyed (*bb*) and 80% homozygous brown-eyed people (*BB*). If that population is under Hardy-Weinberg equilibrium, what will be at equilibrium the percentages of heterozygotes and the other homozygotes?

Percentage of *BB* = 80% = 0.80 = *p*

Percentage of *bb* = 20% = 0.20 = *q*

At Hardy-Weinberg equilibrium, the distribution of three genotypes will be:

$p^2 BB + 2pq Bb + q^2 bb = (0.80)^2 BB + 2(0.80 \times 0.20) Bb + (0.20)^2 bb$

= 0.64 or 64% BB, 0.32 or 32% Bb, and 0.04 or 4% bb

6.4.9   In humans, the gene for brown eyes (B) is completely dominant over the blue (b) such that the individuals of the BB and Bb genotypes are brown eyed and bb are blue eyed. The genes I^A and I^B are codominant with the genotypes $I^A I^A$, $I^A I^B$ and $I^B I^B$ result in the A, B and AB blood types. If 90% of the population is homozygous brown eyed, 10% blue eyed and all the 100% belong to AB blood type, what will be the relative proportions of different genotypes if the population is at Hardy-Weinberg equilibrium?

% of BB =90% = 0.90

% of bb = 10% = 0.10

Distribution of genotypes for eye colour, at Hardy-Weinberg equilibrium will be:

p^2 *BB* + *2pq* *Bb* + q^2 *bb*

= $(0.90)^2$ *BB* + 2 (0.90 × 0.10) *Bb* + $(0.10)^2$ *bb*

= 0.81 or 81% BB, 0.18 or 18% Bb, and 0.01 or 1% bb

Similarly, the distribution of genotypes for blood groups at Hardy-Weinberg equilibrium will be:

p^2 $I^A I^A$ + *2pq* $I^A I^B$ + q^2 $I^B I^B$

= $(0.90)^2$ *BB* + 2 (0.90 × 0.10) *Bb* + $(0.10)^2$ *bb*

= 0.81 or 81% BB, 0.18 or 18% Bb, and 0.01 or 1% bb

6.4.10 In an electrophoresis, two alleles namely PGI-2a and PGI-2b were found affect the electrophoretic mobility of the enzyme; in a total of 57 strains, 35 PGI-2a/ PGI-2a, 19 PGI-2a/ PGI-2b and 3 PGI-2b/ PGI-2b. Calculate the expected numbers of the three genotypes assuming that the genotypes occur in Hardy-Weinberg equilibrium.

6.4.11 In a population of 3100 people, 1101 were found to be MM, 1496 MN and 503 were NN. Calculate the allele frequencies of M and N and the expected numbers of the three genotypic classes.

6.4.12 In a study on 400 people, 230 were found to be Rh^+ and 170 were Rh^-. Calculate the allele frequencies of D (i.e., the allele which in homozygous form results in the Rh^+ phenotype) and d (the allele which in homozygous form results in the Rh^- phenotype; recall that the phenotype Dd is Rh^+). How many of the Rh^+ individuals would be expected to be heterozygous?

6.4.13 In a sampled population, 36% were horned (pp). Using this, calculate the following:

(a) Frequency of horned genotype

(b) Frequency of horned (p) allele

(c) Frequency of polled (P) allele

(d) Frequency of the genotypes PP and Pp

(e) Frequencies of the two possible phenotypes, if 'P' is completely dominant over 'p'.

Answers:

(a) Frequency of the horned (pp) genotype is 36%, as given in the problem itself.

(b) The frequency of 'pp' is 36%, which mean that $q^2 = 0.36$. If $q^2 = 0.36$, then $q = 0.6$ or 60%, again by the definition that gene frequency = square root of genotype frequency.

(c) Since $q = 0.6$ and $p + q = 1$, then $p = 0.4$; the frequency of P is by definition equal to the polled (dominant) gene P. So, the answer is 0.4 or 40%.

(d) The frequency of 'PP' is p^2 and the frequency of Aa is equal to 2pq. So, using the information above, the frequency of PP is 16% (i.e., p^2 is $0.4 \times 0.4 = 0.16$) and Aa is 48% (i.e., $2 \times 0.4 \times 0.6$).

(e) Since 'P' is completely dominant over 'p', the dominant phenotype will appear if either it is homozygous 'PP' or heterozygous 'Pp' genotype. Therefore, the frequency of the dominant phenotype equals the sum of the frequencies of PP and Pp, which is 0.64 or 64% [$(0.4 \times 0.4) + (2 \times 0.6 \times 0.4)$).

6.4.14 In humans, the sickle cell anemia is an autosomal recessive genetic disease. The homozygous-dominant individuals (SS) have normal blood cells that are easily infected with the malarial parasite. Hence, many of these individuals become ill from the parasite infection and may die. The persons homozygous for the sickle cell trait (ss) have the red blood cells, which collapse when deoxygenated, whereas the individuals with heterozygous condition (Ss) suffer from the sickle-shaped RBCs but generally not harmful to the extent that it can cause mortality. The malarial parasites cannot survive in these partially defective RBCs. Hence, the heterozygotes (Ss) survive better than the individuals suffering from severe form of sickle cell anemia (ss).

6.4.15 If 9% of the individuals in a population suffer from sickle cell anemia, what percentage of the population will be more resistant to malaria because they are heterozygous (Ss) for the sickle cell gene?

Ans: Genotype frequency (ss) of sickle cell = $q^2 = 0.09$. Therefore, q = square root of q^2, we get 0.3. Since $q = 0.3$, then the gene frequency of S gene = $p = 1.0 - 0.3 = 0.7$. Hence, the frequency of heterozygous (Ss) carriers = 2 pq = $2 \times 0.7 \times 0.3 = 0.42$ or 42.0%.

6.4.16   A population of 40 guinea pigs undergoing natural selection is reduced to 20 individuals in five generations. At this point, the genotype frequencies are 0.25, 0.50 and 0.25 for the genotypes AA, Aa and aa, respectively. Assume that natural selection continues to act on this population. Is the population in Hardy-Weinberg equilibrium?

6.4.17   In a population of butterflies, the brown colour (B) is dominant over the white (b). If 40% of these flies were white, calculate the percentage of butterflies in the population that are heterozygous and the frequency of homozygous dominant flies. (Answers: 0.47 and 0.14).

6.4.18   In humans, the red skin colour is totally recessive to tan. If a population consists of 396 red and 557 tan individuals, (a) calculate the allele frequencies of each allele, (b) expected genotype frequencies, (c) number of heterozygous individuals, (d) expected phenotype frequencies; and if there are 1245 individuals in a village, how many of them are expected to be red and tan coloured.

Ans:

(a) Total number of individuals = 396 + 557 = 953. Recessive (red) genotype frequency = q^2 = 396/(396 + 557) = 396/953 = 0.416. Therefore, q, the allele frequency of red allele = square root of 0.416 = 0.645. Since p + q = 1, then p must be 1.000 − 0.645 = 0.355.

(b) Expected genotype frequencies of AA = p^2 = $(0.355)^2$ = 0.126; Aa = 2pq = 2 × 0.355 × 0.645 = 0.458; and aa = q^2 = $(0.645)^2$ = 0.416.

(c) Number of heterozygous individuals predicted to be in the population = N × 2pq = 953 × 2 × 0.355 × 0.645 = about 436.

(d) Expected phenotypes of tan skin colour = N × $(p^2 + 2pq)$ = 1245 × $(0.355^2 + 2 × 0.355 × 0.645)$ = 1245 (0.126 + 0.458) = 1245 × 0.584 = 727 and those of red skin are N × q^2 = 1245 × 0.645^2 = 518 or (total number of individuals − number of tan individuals) = 1245 − 727 = 518.

6.4.19   A sample of 1000 individuals was drawn from a large population for blood type and the following results were obtained.

Blood type	Genotype	No. of individuals
M	MM	490
MN	MN	420
N	NN	90

Calculate the frequency of each allele in the population and the probability of each genotype resulting from each potential cross.

6.4.20 Cystic fibrosis is a recessive condition that affects about 1 in 2500 babies in a population. Calculate the frequencies of recessive allele, dominant allele and the percentage of heterozygous individuals (carriers) in the population.

6.4.21 In a population, only "A" and "B" alleles are present in the ABO system; there are no individuals with type "O" blood or with "O" alleles in this population. If 200 people have type A blood; 75 have type AB blood and 25 have type B blood, what are the allelic frequencies of this population (i.e., what are p and q).

6.4.22 The ability to taste PTC is due to a single dominant allele "T". In a sample of 215 individuals, 150 could detect the bitter taste of PTC and 65 could not. Calculate all the potential frequencies.

6.4.23 In a study on blood types in a population, the genotypic distribution among the people sampled was as follows: 1101 MM, 1496 were MN and 503 were NN. Calculate the genotype frequencies of three genotypes; allele frequencies of M and N alleles; expected numbers of the three genotypic classes assuming random mating and using chi-square; determine whether or not this population is in Hardy-Weinberg equilibrium.

Genotype frequencies:

MM = 1101/3100 = 0.356

MN = 1496/3100 = 0.482

NN = 503/3100 = 0.162

Allele frequencies:

Frequency of M allele = $p = p^2 + 1/2(2pq) = 0.356 + 1/2(0.482) = 0.356 + 0.241 = 0.597$

Frequency of N allele = $q = q^2 + 1/2(2pq) = 0.162 + 1/2(0.482) = 0.162 + 0.241 = 0.403$ or $q = (1 - p) = (1.000 - 0.597 = 0.403)$

Expected genotype frequencies (assuming Hardy-Weinberg equilibrium):

MM (p^2) = $(0.597)^2$ = 0.357

MN (2pq) = (2 × 0.597 × 0.403) = 0.481

NN (q^2) = $(0.403)^2$ = 0.162

Sum of the genotypic frequencies = 0.357 + 0.481 + 0.162 = 1.000

Expected number of individuals of each genotype out of the total (1101 + 1496 + 503 = 3100):

No. of MM individuals = N × (p^2) = 3100 × 0.597^2 = 1105

No. of MN individuals = N × (2pq) = 3100 × (2 × 0.597 × 0.403) = 1492

No. of NN individuals = N × (q^2) = 3100 × (0.403^2) = 503

Chi-square test:

H_0 (Null hypothesis): The population is in Hardy-Weinberg equilibrium.

$\chi^2 = \Sigma\,(O - E)^2/E$

= $[(1101 - 1105)^2/1105]$ + $[(1496 - 1492)^2/1492]$ + $[(503 - 503)^2/503]$

= 0.014 + 0.011 + 0.000 = 0.025

χ^2 calculated value at 1 d.f., 5% LS is 3.841.

Conclusion: Since the χ^2 calculated value is less than the χ^2 table value, the null hypothesis is accepted and it is concluded that the population is in Hardy-Weinberg equilibrium (HWE).

6.4.24 In human blood groups, a sample of 100 individuals contained 50 MM, 20 MN and 30 NN individuals. Calculate the frequencies of M and N alleles and test whether this sample is in Hardy-Weinberg equilibrium.

6.4.25 The M-N blood types of humans are under the genetic control of a pair of codominant alleles. In families of six children, where both parents are of blood type MN, what is the chance of finding children of M, 2 of type MN and 1 N?

Parents: MN   ×   MN

Children: 1/4 MM (M-type) 2/4 MN (MN-type) 1/4 NN (N-type)

Probability: 1/4   1/2   1/4

Let k_1 = no. of children of type 'M' required = 3

Let k_2 = no. children of type MN required = 2

Let k_3 = no. of children of 'N' required = 1

$N = \Sigma \, (k_1 + k_2 + k_3) = 3 + 2 + 1 = 6$

$$\text{Principle} = \frac{N!}{k1! \, k2! \, k3!}$$

$$(p_1 + p_2 + p_3)^N = \frac{6!}{3! \, 2! \, 1!} \, (1/4)^3 \, (1/2)^2 \, (1/4)^1 = 15/256$$

Therefore, in a family of six, wherein both the parents are MN, the chance of finding 3 children of type M, 2 of MN and 1 of N type is 15/256.

6.4.26   In a city, the allele frequencies of I^A, I^B and I^O are 0.27, 0.06 and 0.67, respectively. What are the expected frequencies of blood types A, B, AB and O?

6.4.27   The dry type of *ear cerumen* ("wax") is due to homozygosity for a simple Mendelian recessive. Among the people in a country, the frequency of dry-cerumen individuals is 66 percent. What is the frequency of the recessive allele? What is the overall frequency of heterozygotes? Among the individuals with the wet type of cerumen, what is the frequency of heterozygotes? (Assume the population is under Hardy-Weinberg equilibrium).

6.4.28   In an experiment, the amount of polymorphism in the alleles controlling the enzyme *Lactate Dehydrogenase* (*LDH*) in rabbit meat was estimated. A total of 200 bunnies were sampled and the frequencies of the three genotypes AA, Aa and aa were 0.080, 0.280 and 0.640, respectively. From these data, calculate the allele frequencies of A and a alleles in this population. Using the appropriate statistical test, decide whether or not this population is in Hardy-Weinberg equilibrium.

6.4.29   There is an inherited difference in human ability to taste the compound called PTC (phenylthiocarbamide or phenylthiourea). Some people find this compound very bitter; they are called *tasters* for PTC. Others (*nontasters*) find it tasteless. The difference depends on simple Mendelian alternative, in which the allele for taster (T) is dominant to that for nontaster (t). In a population, about 70% were tasters, while the remaining 30% are nontasters. Estimate the frequencies of the taster (T) and nontaster (t) alleles in this population as well as the frequencies of the diploid genotypes.

6.4.30 In a study on human blood groups, it was observed that out of 400 individuals in a population, 230 were Rh⁺ and 170 were Rh⁻. Assuming that this trait (being Rh⁺) is controlled by a dominant allele (D), calculate the allele frequencies of D and d. How many of the Rh⁺ individuals would be expected to be heterozygous?

6.4.31 A randomly mating population has a frequency of Rh⁻ blood types of 16 percent. What is the frequency of the d allele (i.e. Rh⁻ allele)? What is the frequency of D allele (i.e. Rh⁺ allele)? What are the expected genotype frequencies?

6.4.32 Phenylketonuria is a severe form of mental retardation due to an autosomal recessive gene. In a state, about one in every 10,000 children born was affected by the disease. Calculate the frequency of carriers (i.e., heterozygotes).

6.4.33 The I^A allele for the ABO blood groups consists of two subtypes: I^{A1} and I^{A2}, either being considered I^A. In a population about ¾ of the I^A alleles are I^{A1} and ¼ are I^{A2}. Among individuals of genotype $I^A I^O$, what fraction would be expected to be $I^{A1} I^O$? What fraction $I^{A2} I^O$? What would be the expected proportions of $I^{A1} I^{A1}$, $I^{A1} I^{A2}$ and $I^{A2} I^{A2}$ among $I^A I^A$ individuals?

6.4.34 Imagine an autosomal locus with four alleles, A_1, A_2, A_3 and A_4, at frequencies of 0.1, 0.2, 0.3 and 0.4, respectively. Calculate the expected random mating frequencies of all the possible genotypes.

6.4.35 Consider a locus with two alleles (A_1 and A_2) and another locus with three alleles B_1, B_2 and B_3. Let $p_1 = 0.3$, be the allele frequency of A_1 and $q_1 = 0.2$, be that of B_1 and $q_2 = 0.3$ be that of B_2. Calculate the frequencies of all possible gametes, assuming that the loci are in linkage equilibrium.

6.4.36 Suppose the genotypes AA, Aa and aa have frequencies in zygotes of 0.16, 0.48 and 0.36, respectively and relative viabilities of $w11 = 1.0$, $w12 = 0.8$ and $w22 = 0.6$, respectively. Calculate the genotype frequencies in the zygotes in the next generation.

6.4.37 The frequencies in percent of the blood group alleles in a population were computed to be $I^A = 20.62$, $I^B = 7.56$ and $i = 71.83$. What are the expected phenotype frequencies in this population, on the assumption of random mating?

6.4.38 In an aboriginal population, 99 percent of all persons tested were Rh-positive (D⁺). What are the frequencies of the three genotypes

DD, Dd and dd, expected on the assumption of random mating? What proportion of matings in this population would be subject to the risk of having a baby with erythroblastosis due to D incompatibility?

6.4.39   Among a sample of 1000 individuals, the number of persons with each of the MN blood group phenotypes was as follows. M = 298, MN = 489, and N = 213. What are the frequencies of M and N alleles?

6.4.40   In human blood, there are two alleles 'S' and 's' and three distinct phenotypes that can be identified by means of the appropriate reagents. In a sample of 1000 people, the number of people belonging to the three genotypes SS, Ss and ss were 99, 418 and 483, respectively. Calculate the frequency of 'S' and 's' in this population and carry out a χ^2 test. Is there any reason to reject the hypothesis of Hardy-Weinberg proportions in this population?

6.4.41   In plants, the petal colour is controlled by a single gene, whose two alleles B and B_1 are codominant. In a group, 170 plants were homozygous brown, 340 homozygous purple and 21 purple brown. Is this population in Hardy-Weinberg Equilibrium (HWE)? Calculate the Inbreeding coefficient ("F").

(Inbreeding coefficient, F = (Observed heterozygosity – Expected heterozygosity)/ observed heterozygosity)

6.4.42   In a population, before selection consists of 0.5 AA, 0.25 Aa and 025 aa individuals. The relative fitnesses associated with each of these three genotypes are 0.3, 0.5 and 1.0, respectively. Calculate p, the frequency of A before selection and following one round of selection.

6.4.43   Given a population with genotype frequencies of 0.2, 0.2 and 0.6 for the genotypes AA, Aa and aa, respectively, what should be the genotype frequencies assuming Hardy-Weinberg equilibrium?

6.4.44   The B allele is dominant to b allele. The phenotype associated with the former is brown eyes, while blue eyes are the phenotype associated with the latter. The brown eye allele is present in the population at a frequency of 0.2. Given Hardy-Weinberg equilibrium and no differences in allele frequencies between genders, what is the probability that a blue-eyed woman will marry a brown-eyed man?

(Ans: p = 0.2; q = 0.8; p^2 = 0.04; pq = 0.32; q^2 = 0.64; the frequency of brown-eyed people (men or women) is 0.04 + 0.32 = 0.36; the frequency of blue-eyed people (men or women) is 0.64; the probability that a brown-eyed man will marry a blue-eyed woman therefore is 0.36 × 0.64 = 0.23. That is, 23% of all marriages, assuming random marrying, will be between blue-eyed women and brown-eyed men (another 23% will be between blue-eyed men and brown-eyed woman, 41% will consist of all blue-eyed people, and 13% will be between all brown-eyed people).

6.4.45 The hemophilia (failure to clot the blood) in human beings is a sex-linked lethal recessive condition.

 (a) A normal man, whose father is a hemophilic, marries a normal woman with no hemophilia in her ancestry. What is the chance of hemophilia in their children?

  (i) Suppose that this family has two sons, what is the probability that they will both be normal?

  (ii) Suppose that this family has six sons, what is the probability that three will be normal and three hemophilic; two are normal and four hemophilic?

  (iii) If this family is expecting a child, what is the probability that it will be normal? That it will be hemophilic?

 (b) A normal woman, whose father was hemophilic, marries a normal man. What is the chance of hemophilia in their children?

 (c) The parents in the above problem have a normal son. What is the probability that their second son will also be normal?

6.4.46 In garden pea, yellow cotyledon colour is dominant to green and inflated pod shape is dominant to constricted form. When both of these traits considered in self-fertilization hybrid, the progeny appeared in the numbers: 193 green inflated; 184 yellow constricted; 556 yellow inflated; and 61 green constricted. Test the data for independent assortment.

6.4.47 A population of 1000 cattle was found to contain 360 red (RR), 480 roan (Rr) and 160 white (rr) animals. The population mates at random to produce the progeny generation. Assuming the absence of migration, mutation and selection, prove that allelic frequencies remain constant from parental to progeny generation and that the allelic frequencies predict the genotypic frequencies.

6.4.48 In humans, red-green colour blindness is a sex-linked recessive trait. A colour blind male has the genotype X^bY and a normal male has the genotype X^BY, thus for males, the genotype and phenotype frequencies are equal. Females could be X^BX^B (normal), X^BX^b (carrier), or X^bX^b (colour blind), thus the normal Hardy-Weinberg Law applies. If 10% (0.10) of the males are colour blind and 90% (0.90) are normal, then p = 0.90 and q = 0.10 because each male has only one allele for this gene. From this the phenotype frequencies for the females can be calculated: $p^2 = (0.90)^2 = 0.81$ (or 81%) normal, $2pq = 2 \times 0.90 \times 0.10 = 0.18$ (or 18%) carriers and $q^2 = (0.10)^2 = 0.01$ (or 1%) colour blind.

If the frequency of red-green colour blind males in a population is 0.20, what is the frequency of red-green colour blind females in this population? What proportion of the females could have red-green colour blind sons?

6.4.49 The Hardy-Weinberg Law also applies for multiple genes. For example, for a gene with alleles A and a, $p_A + q_a = 1$ and $p^2_A + 2p_Aq_a + q^2_a = 1$ and for some other gene with alleles B and b, $p_B + q_b = 1$ and $p^2_B + 2p_Bq_b + q^2_b = 1$. Note that, assuming these are not linked genes, p_A and q_a are totally unrelated to and independent of p_B and q_b. If, for example, it is desired to find the frequency of AaBb, multiply the frequencies needed $(2p_Aq_a \times 2p_Bq_b)$. If $p_A = 0.2$ (thus $q_a = 0.8$) and $p_B = 0.1$ (thus $q_b = 0.9$), then the probability of AaBb should be $2 \times 0.2 \times 0.8 \times 2 \times 0.1 \times 0.9 = 0.058$.

(a) What will the frequency of the genotype AaBB be at equilibrium if the frequency of a is 0.60 and the frequency of b is 0.20? What genotype will be most frequent in this population?

6.4.50 *Ectrodactyly*, also known as *lobster claw*, is an autosomal recessive condition in humans in which the fingers and toes are fused. Otherwise, individuals with this condition are healthy. Suppose the frequency of ectrodactyly among newborns is approximately 1/10,000 (when the parents are unrelated):

(a) What is the risk of a child with ectrodactyly if the parents are siblings?

If the frequency of ectrodactyly among newborns is 1/10,000 when the parents are unrelated, then the allele frequency (q) of the disease allele (a) is q = (1/10,000) = 0.01, p = 0.99

To estimate the risk of getting an ectrodactyly affected child from a brother–sister mating, we need to calculate the inbreeding coefficient (F) for such a mating:

F = P (homozygous by descent for full siblings) = 1/4

The frequency of homozygous recessives for full sib mating is $q^2 + pq$ (1/4) = $(0.01)^2 + (0.01) (0.99) (1/4)$ = 0.0026 = approximately three in every thousand.

(b) What is the risk of a child with PKU if the parents are second cousins?

F for second cousins is 1/64, so following the same calculations as above:

The frequency of homozygous recessives for second cousin mating is $q^2 + pq$ (1/64) = $(0.01)^2 + (0.01) (0.99) (1/64)$ = 0.00025 = approximately two-three in every ten thousand.

6.4.51 In a large, randomly mating population of giraffes with no movement of individuals in and out of the population and no mutation, the two alleles at one gene, A and a, do not affect survival or reproduction of the giraffes. The two alleles at the other gene, S and B, do affect survival to adulthood by affecting the degree to which giraffes are subject to parasitism by ticks and biting flies. BB individuals have bitter blood, which repels parasites, and survive best. SB individuals have neutral tasting blood and survive 80% as well as do BB individuals. SS individuals have sweet blood and attract parasites; they survive only 4% as well as do BB individuals.

(a) In a population of adult giraffes, the frequency of individuals with the AA genotype is 0.04. Calculate the frequency of individuals with the Aa genotype.

At the A, a gene, the population is in Hardy-Weinberg Equilibrium. So:

Adult Frequency of AA = 0.04 = p^2

Allele frequency of A = p = square root of 0.04 = 0.20

Allele frequency of a = q = 1 – p = 1 – 0.20 = 0.80

Genotype frequency of Aa = 2pq = 2*(0.20)*(0.80) = 0.32

(b) In a population of gametes at the start of a generation, the frequency of the B allele is 0.14. Calculate the frequency of zygotes with the SB genotype:

Allele frequency of B = 0.14 = p

Allele frequency of S = $1 - p = 1 - 0.14 = 0.86$

Zygote genotype frequencies are in Hardy-Weinberg proportions, so:

Genotype frequency of SB in zygotes = $2pq = 2(0.14)(0.86) = 0.24$

(c) Continuing from part (b), calculate the frequency of the adults that survive from the zygotes that have the SB genotype.

$w_{BB} = 1$ $w_{SB} = 0.80$ $w_{as} = 0.04$

wbar = $w_{BB}p^2 + w_{SB}2pq + w_{SS}q^2 = (1)(0.14)^2 + (0.80)(2)(0.14)(0.86) + (0.04)(0.86)^2 = 0.24$

Adult genotype frequencies: Freq(BB) = $w_{BB}p^2$/wbar = $(1)(0.14)^2/0.24 = 0.08$

Freq(SB) = $w_{SB}2pq$/wbar = $(0.80)(2)(0.14)(0.86)/0.24 = 0.80$

Freq(SS) = $w_{SS}q^2$/wbar = $(0.04)(0.86)^2/0.24 = 0.12$

(d) Continuing from part (c), calculate the frequency of the B allele in the gametes that will produce the next generation.

Allele frequencies produced by adults to start the next generation:

Frequency of B = Freq(BB) + (1/2) Freq(SB) = $0.08 + (1/2)(0.8) = 0.48$

6.4.52 Consider two genes in a large, randomly mating population of turtles with no movement of individuals in and out of the population and no mutation. The two alleles at one gene, L and M, do not affect fitness. The two alleles at the other gene, T and t, do affect fitness – they affect the thickness of turtle shells, and the degree to which they are protected from predation. TT individuals have thick shells, which repel predators, and survive best. Tt individuals have medium shell thickness and survive 88% as well as do TT individuals. tt individuals have thin shells and are easy for predators to eat; they survive only 14% as well as do TT individuals.

(a) In a population of adult turtles, the frequency of individuals with the MM genotype is 0.06. Calculate the frequency of individuals with the LM genotype.

Since there are no fitness differences, this gene is in Hardy-Weinberg Equilibrium.

Freq. MM = $0.06 = p^2$

Freq. M = p = the square root of p^2 = the square root of 0.06 = 0.24

Freq. L = q = $1 - p = 1 - 0.24 = 0.76$

Freq. LM = $2pq = 2(0.24)(0.76) = 0.36$

(b) In a population of gametes at the start of a generation, the frequency of the t allele is 0.23. Calculate the frequency of zygotes with the Tt genotype.

Freq. t = $0.23 = q$; Freq. T = $p = 1 - 0.23 = 0.77$

Zygote genotype frequencies are in Hardy-Weinberg proportions, so:

Freq. Tt = $2pq = 2(0.77)(0.23) = 0.35$

(c) Continuing from part (b), calculate the frequency of the adults that survive from the zygotes that have the Tt genotype.

To calculate adult genotype frequencies, we need to know the relative fitnesses of the genotypes. These are:

TT survives the best, and the highest relative fitness is always 1, so $w_{TT} = 1$

Tt survives 88% as well as TT, so $w_{Tt} = 0.88$

tt survives 14% as well as TT, so $w_{tt} = 0.14$

Now, to calculate adult genotype frequencies, the first step is to calculate the average population fitness, wbar:

wbar = $w_{TT}p^2 + w_{Tt}2pq + w_{tt}q^2$

wbar = $(1)(0.77)^2 + (0.88)(2)(0.77)(0.23) + (0.14)(0.23)^2 = 0.91$

Freq. Tt = $w_{Tt}2pq$ / wbar = $(0.88)(2)(0.77)(0.23) / 0.91 = 0.34$

(d) Continuing from part (c), calculate the frequency of the t allele in the gametes that will produce the next generation.

To calculate the frequency of t, we need to use the formula

Freq. t = Freq. tt + (1/2) Freq. Tt

To use this, we first calculate Freq. Tt = $w_{tt}q^2$ / wbar = $(0.14)(0.23)^2 / 0.91 = 0.0081$

Freq. t = Freq. tt + (1/2) Freq. Tt = $(0.0081) + (1/2)(0.34) = 0.18$

6.4.53 You have sampled a population in which you know that the percentage of the homozygous recessive genotype (aa) is 36%. Using that 36%, calculate the following:

(a) The frequency of the "aa" genotype

(b) The frequency of the "a" allele

(c) The frequency of the "A" allele

(d) The frequencies of the genotypes "AA" and "Aa"

(e) The frequencies of the two possible phenotypes if "A" is completely dominant over "a"

6.4.54 Sickle cell anemia is an interesting genetic disease. Normal homozygous individuals (SS) have normal blood cells that are easily infected with the malarial parasite. Thus, many of these individuals become very ill from the parasite and many die. Individuals homozygous for the sickle-cell trait (ss) have red blood cells that readily collapse when deoxygenated. Although malaria cannot grow in these red blood cells, individuals often die because of the genetic defect. However, individuals with the heterozygous condition (Ss) have some sickling of red blood cells, but generally not enough to cause mortality. In addition, malaria cannot survive well within these "partially defective" red blood cells. Thus, heterozygotes tend to survive better than either of the homozygous conditions. If 9% of an African population is born with a severe form of sickle cell anemia (ss), what percentage of the population will be more resistant to malaria because they are heterozygous (Ss) for the sickle-cell gene?

6.4.55 There are 100 students in a class. Ninety-six did well in the course whereas four blew it totally and received a grade of F; sorry. In the highly unlikely event that these traits are genetic rather than environmental, if these traits involve dominant and recessive alleles, and if the four (4%) represent the frequency of the homozygous recessive condition, please calculate the following:

(a) The frequency of the recessive allele

(b) The frequency of the dominant allele

(c) The frequency of heterozygous individuals

6.4.56 (a) Suppose that at a two-allele locus in a random-mating diploid population, we find 32% of the individuals to be of the aa phenotype. What fraction of the individuals are Aa?

(b) In a population where the frequency of a is 0.4, what proportion of aa individuals have neither parent aa? One parent aa? Both parents aa? Assume that both parents and offspring were produced by random mating.

6.4.57 Suppose there are two populations that have genotype frequencies of AA Aa aa as 0.64 0.32 and 0.04 in population I and 0.09 0.42 0.49 in population II, respectively. If a researcher draws a very large sample, thinking it is coming from a single population, but it is actually composed of individuals, two-third of whom came from population I and one-third from population II,

(i) Are the two original populations each in Hardy-Weinberg proportions?

(ii) If these individuals are simply collected together, but have no time to interbreed,   what will the genotype frequencies in the sample expected to be?

(iii) What will the gene frequencies be in that sample?

(iv) If we mistakenly assume that the sample is from a single random-mating population, assume that it is in Hardy-Weinberg proportions, and use the sample gene frequency, what proportion of heterozygotes will we expect to see?

6.4.58 A locus has three alleles, B', B and b. B' is completely dominant to B, and both of these are completely dominant to b. What are the frequencies of the three alleles in a random-mating population which has these phenotype frequencies: 50% B'-, 30% B-, and 20% bb?

6.4.59 When we sample 100 individuals from a random mating population, we observe 63AA, 27 Aa and 10 aa. Put 95% confidence limits on the frequency of A. What have you had to assume?

6.4.60 Among 100 individuals, we observe 10 aa(s). Assuming random mating, how do you place 95% confidence limits on the frequency of A?

6.4.61 We sample 200 individuals from a diploid population and find 89 AA, 57 Aa, and 54 aa individuals. Test the hypothesis that this is a sample from a population that is Hardy-Weinberg proportions.

6.4.62 Within a population of butterflies, the color brown (B) is dominant over the color white (b). And, 40% of all butterflies are white. Given this simple information, which is something that is very likely to be on an exam, calculate the following:

(a) The percentage of butterflies in the population that are heterozygous

(b) The frequency of homozygous-dominant individuals

6.4.63   A very large population of randomly mating laboratory mice contains 35% white mice. White coloring is caused by the double recessive genotype, "aa". Calculate allelic and genotypic frequencies for this population.

6.4.64   In a sample of 1,000 individuals from a large population for the MN blood group, the following blood types were noted.

Blood type	Genotype	Number of individuals	Resulting frequency
M	MM	490	0.49
MN	MN	420	0.42
N	NN	90	0.09

Using the data provide above, calculate the following:

(a) The frequency of each allele in the population

(b) Supposing the matings are random, the frequencies of the matings

(c) The probability of each genotype resulting from each potential cross

6.4.65   Cystic fibrosis is a recessive condition that affects about 1 in 2,500 babies in a population. Please calculate the following.

(a) The frequency of the recessive allele in the population

(b) The frequency of the dominant allele in the population

(c) The percentage of heterozygous individuals (carriers) in the population

6.4.66   Three codominant alleles of a single gene determine different forms of an enzyme in a human population. In one sample of 35 individuals, the following data were recorded. Estimate the frequencies of A_1, A_2 and A_3 alleles in this sample.

Genotype	A_1A_1	A_1A_2	A_2A_2	A_2A_3	A_3A_3	A_1A_3
No. of individuals	2	5	12	10	5	1

(Ans: The number of alleles of each type are: A1 = 2 + 2 + 5 + 1 = 10; A2 = 5 + 12 + 12 + 10 = 39; A3 = 10 + 5 + 5 + 1 = 21. The total number of alleles is 70, so the allele frequencies are A1 = 10/70 = 0.14; A2 = 39/70 = 0.56; A3 = 21/70 = 0.30)

6.4.67 The DNA from 100 unrelated individuals in a village was digested with the restriction enzyme *HindIII* and the resulting fragments were fractionated and probed with a sequence for a particular gene. Four fragment lengths that hybridized with the probe were observed namely, 5.7, 6.0, 6.2 and 6.5 kb, where each fragment is a different restriction enzyme allele. The following figure shows the gel patterns observed; the number of individuals with each gel pattern is shown in the top. Estimate the allele frequencies of the four restriction enzymes.

Allele size (kb)	No. of individuals									
	9	21	12	15	18	6	6	7	5	1
6.5	----	----		----		----				
6.2		----	----		----			----		
6.0				----	----	----			----	
5.7							----	----	----	----

(Ans: Allele 5.7 frequency = 2 (6 + 7 + 5 + 1)/2 * 100 = 0.10
Allele 6.0 frequency = 2 (15 + 18 + 6 + 5)/2 * 100 = 0.25
Allele 6.2 frequency = 2 (21 + 12 + 18 + 7)/2 * 100 = 0.35
Allele 6.5 frequency = 2 (9 + 21 + 15 + 6)/2 * 100 = 0.30)

PRACTICAL NO. 7

7.1 CALCULATION OF THE EFFECT OF SELECTION ON CHANGE IN GENE FREQUENCY

A large, random mating population is stable with respect to gene frequencies and genotype frequencies in the absence of the agencies tending to change the genetic properties. There are two sorts of processes which change gene frequency, and consequently the genotype frequencies are changed. The 'systematic processes' change the gene frequency in a manner predictable both in amount and direction. The systematic processes include the migration, mutation and selection. The 'dispersive process' arise in small population from the effects of sampling and is predictable in amount but not in direction.

Selection may be defined as the differential rates of reproduction of different genotypes in a population. When the differential reproduction is consequence of natural factors or the environment, it is called *natural selection*. But when it is brought about by human efforts, it is termed as *artificial selection*. Selection may operate on gametes or the haploid (n) phase – *gametic selection* or the diploid (2n) phase – zygotic selection.

The reproduction rates of different genotypes are expressed relative to that of the genotype having the highest reproduction rate; this relative value is called fitness value or selective value or adaptive value and it is denoted by 'W', which can be estimated as:

$W = R_i/R_h$, where, R_i is the rate of reproduction of the concerned genotype, and R_h is the rate of reproduction of that genotype, which has the highest reproduction rate. The fitness varies from 0 to 1.

Gametic selection: When selection acts on gametes or on the haploid phase of life cycle, it is called gametic selection. In most fungi, the main part of life cycle is haploid; therefore, the selection in these organisms will be gametic. In some higher organisms, which are normally diploid, gametes, having certain genotypes are known to have differential survival or capability for effecting fertilization; such a phenomenon is called *segregation distortion* or *meiotic drive*.

Zygotic selection: Higher organisms are diploid and their haploid phase is only short lived and totally dependent on the diploid phase. In these organisms, selection operates on the zygotes and the diploid phase.

The zygotic selection may be (i) against the recessive phenotype, (ii) against the dominant phenotype and (iii) in favour of the heterozygotes.

When a gene is subject to selection, its frequency in the offspring will not be the same as in the parents, since parents of different genotypes contribute genes unequally to the next generation. The proportionate contribution of offspring to the next generation is called the 'fitness' of the individual. Thus, the selection causes a change in gene frequency, and consequently the genotype frequency.

Selection may operate either through the reduced fertility among the parents or the reduced viability in the offspring. In either case, the genotype selected against make a smaller contribution of gametes to form zygotes in the next generation.

The strength of selection is expressed as the 'coefficient of selection', which is defined as the proportionate reduction in the gametic contribution by a genotype in comparison to a standard genotype, usually the most favoured. For example, if $s = 0.1$, it indicated that for every 100 zygotes produced by the favoured genotype, only 90 are produced by the genotype selected against.

Change of gene frequency under selection

Let the two alleles A_1 and A_2 at a locus A in a large, random mating population have the initial gene frequencies p and q, respectively. A_1 being completely dominant over A_2 and the coefficient of selection against recessive genotype A_2A_2 be s. The homozygous dominant and heterozygous genotypes have fitness value of one, while the homozygous recessives have the fitness of $(1 - s)$. Then, the proportionate contribution of each genotype to the next generation in the form of gametes may be obtained by multiplying the initial frequency with the fitness value, as shown below.

	Genotypes			Total
	A_1A_1	A_1A_2	A_2A_2	
Initial frequency	p^2	$2pq$	q^2	1
Relative frequency	1	1	$(1 - s)$	
Gametic contribution to next generation	$p^2 \times 1$ $= p^2$	$2pq \times 1$ $= 2pq$	$q^2 (1 - s)$	$p^2 + 2pq + q^2 (1 - s) = (1 - sq^2)$

$p^2 + 2pq + q^2 (1 - s) = p^2 + 2pq + q^2 - q^2s = (1 - sq^2)$ because, $p^2 + 2pq + q^2 = 1$

The total gametic contribution to the next generation will never be unity or 100% since there is a proportionate loss of sq^2 due to selection. To get the frequency of A_2 genes in the offspring generation, we need to take the gametic contribution of A_2A_2 individuals and half the contribution of A_1A_2 individuals and divide by the total. Thus, the gene frequency of A_2 gene (q) in the offspring will be:

$$q_1 = \frac{q^2(1-s) + \frac{1}{2}(2pq)}{(1-sq^2)}$$

$$= \frac{q^2 - sq^2 + pq}{(1-sq^2)} = \frac{-q^2 - sq^2 + (1-q)q}{(1-sq^2)} \quad \text{since } p = (1-q)$$

$$\frac{q^2 - sq^2 + q - q^2}{(1-sq^2)} = \frac{sq^2 + q}{(1-sq^2)} = \frac{q(1-sq)}{(1-sq^2)}$$

The change in gene frequency of A_2 gene per generation due to selection is equal to the gene frequency in offspring generation minus initial gene frequency.

$$= q_1 - q$$

$$= \frac{q(1-sq)}{(1-sq^2)} - q$$

$$\frac{q - sq^2 - q(1-sq^2)}{(1-sq^2)}$$

$$= \frac{q^2 - sq^2 - q + sq^2}{(1-sq^2)} = \frac{-sq^2 + sq}{(1-sq^2)} = \frac{-sq^2(1-q)}{(1-sq^2)}$$

Thus, the effect of selection on gene frequency depends on the coefficient of selection (s) and the initial gene frequency, i.e. q.

CLASS WORK

1. In a population of goats, the hornless condition caused y the homozygous recessive genotype, hh is undesirable and in contrast, the horned condition (HH, Hh) is desirable. The frequencies of HH, Hh and hh genotypes in a flock were 0.36, 0.48 and 0.16, respectively. If it is decided to cull 50% of all hornless animals from the flock, calculate the allelic frequencies in the next generation and find out the change in gene frequency of h gene (q) after one generation of selection.

Genotype	Genotype frequency	Fitness (W) or Coefficient of selection	Gametic contribution (Frequency × fitness)
HH	0.36 (p^2)	$1 - 0 = 1.0$	$1.0 \times 0.36 = 0.36$
Hh	0.48 (2pq)	$1 - 0 = 1.0$	$1.0 \times 0.48 = 0.48$
Hh	0.16 (q^2)	$1 - 0.5 = 0.5$	$0.5 \times 0.16 = 0.08$
Total gametic contribution to next generation =			0.92

Frequency of h gene (q) $= 1 - p = 1.000 - 0.652 = 0.348$

Frequency of h gene prior to selection (q_0) $= \sqrt{q^2} = \sqrt{0.16} = 0.4$

Change of gene frequency (Δq) $= q_0 - q = 0.400 - 0.348 = 0.052$ or 5.2%

2. A locus has two alleles T and t with the frequencies of 0.65 and 0.35, respectively. The homozygous recessives have fitness value of 0.3, while the other two genotypes have the fitness values of 1.0 each. If the individuals of this population interbreed to produce the next generation, what is the frequency of T gene in the next generation?

Given that $p = 0.65$, $q = 0.35$ and $s = 0.7$

Change in gene frequency of t gene due to selection against tt genotype in one generation =

$= (spq^2)/(1 - sq^2) = (0.3 \times 0.65 \times 0.35^2)/[1 - (0.3 \times 0.35^2)]$

$= -0.0248$

In the next generation, the frequency of recessive t gene will be $0.3500 - 0.0248 = 0.3252$

Therefore, the frequency of dominant allele, T will be $1 - 0.3252 = 0.6748$.

HOME WORK

7.1.1   (a) The coefficients of selection for the AA and aa genotypes are 0.1 and 0.0, respectively. There is complete dominance of the A allele over the a allele. What are the fitnesses of the three genotypes?

$W_{AA} = 0.9$, $W_{Aa} = 0.9$, $W_{aa} = 1.0$

(b) If 40 out of a hundred individuals with the AA and Aa genotypes survive to reproductive age and 80 out of 100 individuals with the aa genotype survive to reproductive age what are the fitnesses of the three genotypes?

$W_{AA} = 0.4/0.8 = 0.5$, $W_{Aa} = 0.4/0.8 = 0.5$, $W_{aa} = 0.8/0.8 = 1.0$

7.1.2   The yellow fat character in sheep is responsible for the failure to oxidize the fat-soluble plant pigment xanthophyll, and this trait is undesirable from the meat purchase point of view. In a large random mating population of Nellore sheep under Hardy-Weinberg equilibrium, the number of animals homozygous recessive for yellow fat (yy) were 9%, while the heterozygous carriers (Yy) and the non-yellow fat (homozygous dominants) individuals constituted 42% and 49%, respectively. Since the yellow fat is undesirable, selection is undertaken against these animals by culling 50% of them. Calculate initial frequency of yellow fat gene (q) and frequency of this allele after one generation of selection (q_1).

7.1.3   In a population under selection, initial gene frequency of a recessive gene was 0.2 and the coefficient of selection against the homozygous recessive genotype was 0.3. Calculate the change in gene frequency of a gene for one generation of selection.

7.1.4   In a large random mating population under selection, the frequency of a recessive gene was 0.4 and coefficient of selection against recessive genotype was 0.6. Calculate the gene frequency of recessive gene in the offspring generation. Also find out the change in gene frequency per generation.

7.2 CALCULATION OF THE EFFECT OF MIGRATION ON CHANGE IN GENE FREQUENCY

Inter change of the individuals between populations is called migration. Migration causes a change in the gene frequency, genetic mean and the variance of a population. Suppose that a large population consists of a proportion, m, of immigrants in each generation and the remaining proportion $(1 - m)$ being the natives. Let the frequency of a certain gene be q_m among the immigrants and q_0 among the natives. Then, the frequency of the gene in mixed population (q_1) will be:

$$q_1 = mq_m + (1 - m) q_0$$
$$= mq_{m} + q_0 - mq_0$$
$$= m (q_m - q_0) + q_0$$

The change in gene frequency, q, brought about by one generation of immigration will be the difference between the gene frequency before immigration and gene frequency after immigration.

$$q = q_1 - q_0$$
$$= m (q_m - q_0) + q_0 - q_0$$
$$= m (q_m - q_0)$$

Thus, the rate of change of gene frequency in a population subject to immigration depends on the proportion migrated and the difference of gene frequency between immigrants and natives.

CLASS WORK

1. A population consists of 10% of the immigrants in each generation. The gene frequency of a gene before migration is 0.3 and the frequency of the same gene after migration is 0.5. Calculate the gene frequency in the mixed population after immigration and change in gene frequency per generation.

Proportion migrated (m)	=	10% = 0.1
Gene frequency before immigration (q_0)	=	0.3
Gene frequency after immigration (q_m)	=	0.5
Gene frequency in mixed population (q_1)	=	$m (q_m - q_0) + q_0$
	=	0.10 (0.5 − 0.3) + 0.3
	=	0.32

$$
\begin{aligned}
\text{Change of gene frequency } (\Delta\, q) \quad &= \quad m\,(q_m - q_0) \\
&= \quad 0.10\,(0.5 - 0.3) \\
&= \quad 0.02
\end{aligned}
$$

HOME WORK

7.2.1   In a native population, 2.6% of the individuals had type A blood, 0.0% have type B, 0.0% have type AB, and 97.4% have type O. Thus, for this population, $p_A = 0.013$, $q_B = 0$ and $r_O = 0.987$. In an exotic population, 42.4% had type A blood, 8.3% have type B, 1.4% have type AB, and 47.9% have type O, so $p_A = 0.250$, $q_B = 0.050$, and $r_O = 0.692$. Suppose, if there are 200 individuals in the first population and 30 have migrated from second population into the first one, and they intermarried, what would be the change in the allele frequencies?

7.2.2   In an island, in a population of 150 individuals, the frequency of a dominant allele A was 0.80. A migrant group of 50 individuals in which frequency of A is 0.2 join the island population to form a combined population of 200 individuals. What will be the frequency of A gene in the next generation?

7.2.3   The frequency of a gene in native population is 0.309. The frequency of this gene among the immigrants is 0.70. The immigrants constituted of 5% of mixed population. What will be the gene frequency in mixed population following immigration?

7.2.4   The frequency of wire-haired texture (dominant, W) in two different groups of dogs was 0.25 and 0.60. Calculate the proportion to be migrated to double the frequency of W allele in the first kennel by introducing a sample of dogs from the second population.

7.2.5   The gene frequency of skin pigmentation in a group of mice was 0.30 in natives and 0.70 in a migrant population. If some animals were migrated into the second population to make up 10% of the aggregate population, calculate the allelic frequency in mixed population and change in gene frequency due to migration.

7.2.6   In two cattle populations, the frequency of horned gene (p) and number of individuals are given below.

	Population I	Population II
Frequency of horned gene (q)	0.10	0.60
Number of animals	600	800

7.2.7   A random sample of 200 animals from population I migrated to population II and interbred. Calculate (a) the frequency of recessive allele in mixed population and (b) change in frequency of recessive gene due to migration.

7.2.8   A population of 80 squirrels resides on campus, and the frequency of the Est[1] allele among these squirrels is 0.70. Another population of squirrels is found in a nearby woods, and there the frequency of the Est[1] allele is 0.50. During a severe winter, 20 of the squirrels from the woods population migrate to campus in search of food and join the campus population. What will be the frequency of the Est[1] allele in the campus population in the spring?

7.2.9   In a population of 1000 cows, the frequency of polled gene was 0.2. If 100 bulls from another population in which the frequency of polled gene is 0.6 are migrated. Then calculate the gene frequency of polled gene in the migrated population and change in gene frequency per generation.

7.2.10 In a herd of 600 cattle, the gene frequency of black coat color is 0.6. 30 bulls were immigrated into this herd from a population, in which the gene frequency of black gene was 0.25. Calculate the gene frequency of black coat colour in the mixed population and change in the gene frequency of black coat colour in the gene frequency.

7.3 CALCULATION OF THE EFFECT OF MUTATION ON CHANGE IN GENE FREQUENCY

The effect of mutation on the genetic properties of the population differs depending upon whether the mutational event is non-recurrent (rare and unique) or recurrent. The non-recurrent mutation is of little importance as a cause of change of gene frequency. In recurrent mutation, the mutational event recurs regularly with a characteristic frequency and causes change in gene frequency.

Suppose that there are two alleles A_1 and A_2 at a locus in a population with initial gene frequencies p_0 and q_0, respectively. A_1 gene mutates to A_2 gene at a rate 'u' per generation (i.e., u is the proportion of all A_1 genes which mutate to A_2) and A_2 mutates to A_1 at a rate 'v'. After one generation, there is a gain of A_2 genes equal to up_0 due to mutation in A_1 to A_2 direction and a loss equal to vq_0 due to mutation in A_2 to A_1 direction. Therefore, the change in gene frequency of A_2 gene in one generation is:

$$q = up_0 - vq_0$$

Similarly, the change in gene frequency of A_1 gene in one generation is:

$q = -up + vq$ (since the gene frequency of A_1 genes reduce at the rate of u, therefore, it is −up and by reverse mutation, frequency of A_1 increases, it is +vq). This situation leads to equilibrium in gene frequency, at which there is no further change in gene frequency. The point of equilibrium can be found by equating the change in gene frequency to zero.

$$p = up - vq = 0$$
$$up = vq$$

Therefore, q = equilibrium value for A_2 allele = up/v

$$q = \frac{u(1-q)}{v}$$
$$= \frac{u - uq}{v}$$
$$= vq = u - uq$$

Therefore, $uq + vq = u$; $q(u + v) = u$

$$\text{Hence, } q = \frac{u}{(u + v)}$$

Similarly, equilibrium value for A1 allele will be:

$$p = \frac{v}{(u + v)}$$

Thus, the effect of selection on gene frequency depends on the coefficient of selection (s) and the initial gene frequency, i.e. q.

CLASS WORK

In a population under random mating, the initial gene frequencies of A_1 and A_2 genes are 0.4 and 0.6, respectively. The mutation rate from A_1 to A_2 was 6 per thousand and the reverse mutation rate from A_2 to A_1 gene was one per ten thousand. Calculate the change in gene frequency due to mutation in one generation and also calculate the gene frequency at equilibrium.

$p = 0.4$, $q = 06$, $u = 6/1000 = 0.006$, $v = 1/10,000 = 0.0001$

Change in gene frequency of A_2 gene $= up - vq$

$$= (0.006 \times 0.4) - (0.0001 \times 0.6)$$
$$= 0.0024 - 0.00006$$
$$= 0.00234$$

Gene frequencies at equilibrium:

(a) Gene frequency of A_2 gene $(q) = u/(u + v) = 0.006/(0.006 + 0.0001)$
    $= 0.984$
(b) Gene frequency of A_1 gene $(p) = v/(u + v) = 0.001/(0.006 + 0.0001)$
    $= 0.016$

HOME WORK

7.3.1   In a large random mating population under selection, the frequency of a recessive gene is 0.4 and the coefficient of selection against the recessive genotype was 0.6. Calculate the gene frequency of recessive gene in the offspring generation and also find out the change in gene frequency per generation.

7.3.2   In a population of 1000 cows, the frequency of polled gene is 0.2. If 100 bulls from another population in which the frequency of polled gene is 0.6 are migrated, then calculate the gene frequency of polled gene in mixed population and change in gene frequency per generation.

7.3.3   In cattle, polled condition is dominant over the horned. If the gene frequency of horned gene (p) is 0.2 and the coefficient of selection against the horned condition is 0.5, what will be the gene frequency in offspring generation and what will be the change in gene frequency in one generation of selection?

7.3.4   In a herd of 600 cattle, the gene frequency of black coat colour is 0.6. 30 bulls were immigrated into this herd from a population, in which the gene frequency of black gene was 0.25. Calculate the gene frequency of black coat colour in the mixed population and find out the change in gene frequency after immigration.

7.3.5   In a population, the initial gene frequency of a dominant gene (A) = p_0 and that of its recessive allele (a) = q_0. The rate of mutation from A to a (u) is 15 in 10,000, while the rate of reverse mutation from a to A (v) is 1 in 10,000. Calculate the change in gene frequency in one generation and the gene frequency of A and a genes at equilibrium point, when (a) $p_0 = 0.9$ and $q_0 = 0.1$ and (b) $p_0 = 0.5$ and $q_0 = 0.5$.

PRACTICAL NO. 8

8.1 COMPUTATION OF POPULATION MEAN

The value observed when a trait is measured on an individual is the phenotypic value of that individual. The phenotypic value is attributable to the influence of genotype (G) and environment (E). Population mean refers to the mean phenotypic or genotypic values of the population.

Consider a single locus with two alleles A_1 and A_2 and the genotypic value of one homozygote (A_1A_1) +a, the other homozygote (A_2A_2) −a and that of the heterozygote (A_1A_2) d. The value of heterozygote, d, depends on the degree of dominance. If there is no dominance, d = 0; if A_1 is dominant over A_2, d is positive; and if A_2 is dominant over A_1, d is negative. If the dominance is complete, d is equal to +a or −a; and if there is overdominance, d is greater than +a or less than −a.

Let the gene frequencies of A_1 and A_2 alleles be p and q, respectively. The population mean (M) can be calculated as per the following table.

Genotype	Frequency	Genotypic value	Frequency × value
A_1A_1	p^2	+ a	$+p^2a$
A_1A_2	2pq	d	2pqd
A_2A_2	q^2	−a	$-q^2a$

$$
\begin{aligned}
\text{Population mean (M)} &= p^2a + 2pqd - q^2a \\
&= a\,(p^2 - q^2) + 2pqd \\
&= a\,(p + q)\,(p - q) + 2pqd \\
&= a\,(p - q) + 2pqd, \text{ since } (p + q) = 1
\end{aligned}
$$

The sum of values × frequencies is the men value of the population. This population mean refers to both the mean genotypic value and the mean phenotypic value of the population. The term a (p − q) is attributable to the homozygotes and 2pqd to heterozygotes. If there is no dominance, d = 0 and the value of pqd will be zero.

Therefore, the population mean (M) is:

$$
\begin{aligned}
M &= a\,(p - q) \\
&= a\,(1 - q) - q \text{ since } p = (1 - q)
\end{aligned}
$$

$$= a(1 - q - q)$$
$$= a(1 - 2q)$$

If the dominance is complete (d = a), then the mean is proportional to the square of gene frequency, i.e. $M = a(1 - 2q^2)$.

CLASS WORK

In mice, a recessive gene known as '*pygmy*' reduces the body size. The average body weight of mice of three genotypes (genotypic values) at 6 weeks of age were Pg Pg = 14 g, Pg pg = 12 g and pg pg = 6 g. The mid-point between two homozygotes is $14 + 6 = 20/2 = 10$ on the scale of values assigned as shown below.

	Pg Pg	Pg pg	pg pg
Genotype			
	14	10	6

Genotypic value, $+ a = 14 - 10 = 4$; $d = 12 - 10 = 2$; $-a = 6 - 10 = -4$

Suppose that the pg gene was present at a frequency (q) of 0.1. Then $p = 1 - q = 1 - 0.1 = 0.9$. The population mean can be calculated as:

$$
\begin{aligned}
M &= a(p - q) + 2pqd \\
&= 4(0.9 - 0.1) + 2(0.9 \times 0.2 \times 2) \\
&= 4(0.8) + 2(0.18) \\
&= 3.56
\end{aligned}
$$

The mean value is, however, measured from mid-homozygote point, which is 10. Therefore, the actual value of the population mean is $3.56 + 10 = 13.56$ g.

8.2 AVERAGE EFFECT

Average effect of a gene is the mean deviation from the population mean of the individuals, which received that gene from one parent; and the gene received from the other parent having come at random from the population.

The average effect can be regarded as the average effect of a gene substitution. The average effect of a gene is a property of the population as well as of the gene and it depends upon the gene frequency. The average effect of a gene will be small, when the frequency of recessive gene is low and large, when it is high.

Consider a locus with two alleles A_1 and A_2 with the frequencies p and q, respectively. If the gametes carrying A_1 unite at random with the gametes from the population, the genotype frequency of A_1A_1 will be pa and that of A_1A_2 will be q. The genotypic value of A_1A_1 and A_1A_2 is pq + qd. The difference between this mean value and the population mean is the average effect of the gene A_1, which may be computed as follows:

The population mean (M) = a (p − q) + 2pqd

$$
\begin{aligned}
\alpha_1 &= \text{Average effect of } A_1 \text{ gene} \\
&= [pa + qd] - [a (p - q) + 2pqd] \\
&= pa + qd - ap + aq - 2pqd \\
&= qd + aq - 2pqd \text{ by cancelling out +pa and } -ap \\
&= q [d + a - 2pd] \text{ by taking q as common} \\
&= q [a + d - 2pd] \text{ by re arranging} \\
&= q [a + d (1 - 2p)] \text{ by taking d as common} \\
&= q [a + d (p + q - 2p)] \text{ as 1 is replaced by p + q since p + q = 1} \\
&= q [a + d (q - p)] \text{ by cancelling out one +p and } -p \\
&= q [a + d (q - p)]
\end{aligned}
$$

Similarly, the average effect of the gene A_2 is computed as:

$$\alpha_2 = -p [a + d (q - p)]$$

CLASS WORK

Consider the pygmy (pg) gene in a population of mice, in which the genotypic values of Pg Pg = a = 4g and Pg pg = d = 2 g. If the gene frequency of pg gene is 0.1, then the average effect of substituting Pg gene for pg gene (α_1) would be:

$$\alpha_1 = q [a + d (q - p)]$$
$$= 0.1 [4 + 2 (0.1 - 0.9)] \text{ by substituting the values}$$
$$= 0.1 [4 - 1.60]$$
$$= 0.24$$

Similarly, the average effect of substituting pg gene for Pg gene (α_2) would be:

$$\alpha_2 = -p [a + d (q - p)]$$
$$= -0.9 [4 + 2 (0.1 - 0.9)]$$
$$= -0.9 [4 - 1.6]$$
$$= -2.16$$

The average effect of gene substitution (α) will be:

$$= a + d (q - p)$$
$$= 4 + 2 (0.1 - 0.9) \text{ by substituting the values of a, d, q and p}$$
$$= 2.4$$

Genotypic value (G) of $A_1 A_1$ genotype is computed as:

$$= 2q (\alpha - qd)$$
$$= 2 \times 0.1 (2.4 - (0.1 \times 2)) \text{ by substituting the values}$$
$$= 0.44$$

Genotypic value of $A_1 A_2$ genotype is:

$$= (q - p) \alpha + 2pqd$$
$$= -1.56 \text{ by substituting the values}$$

Genotypic value of $A_2 A_2$ genotype is:

$$= -2p (\alpha + pd)$$
$$= -7.56$$

8.3 BREEDING VALUE

The value of an individual judged by the mean value of its progeny is called the breeding value of the individual. It can be defined as the sum of the average effects of the genes it carries, the summation being made over the pair of alleles at each locus and over all loci. Breeding value is the property of the individual as well as population, from which its mates are drawn. Breeding value may be expressed in absolute units but usually it is expressed as the deviation from the population mean. For a single locus with two alleles A_1 and A_2, the breeding values of these genotypes are the following:

Genotype	Breeding value
A_1A_1	$2\alpha_1 = 2q\alpha$
A_1A_2	$\alpha_1 + \alpha_2 = (q - p)\alpha$
A_2A_2	$2\alpha_2 = -2p\alpha$

Example

Consider the pygmy gene effect on the population, as described in the above example.

q = gene frequency of pg gene = 0.1

α = average effect of gene substitution = 2.4

M = population mean = 13.56 g

Then, the breeding values of three genotypes are

Genotype	Breeding value (A)
Pg Pg	$2q\alpha = 2 \times 0.1 \times 2.4 = +0.48$
Pg pg	$(q - p)\alpha = (0.1 - 0.9) \times 2.4 = 1.92$
pg pg	$-2p\alpha = -2 \times 0.9 \times 2.4 = -4.32$

8.4 DOMINANCE DEVIATION

When a single locus is under consideration, the difference between the genotypic value (G) and breeding value (A) of a genotype is known as dominance deviation (D). $G = A + D$ and therefore, $D = G - A$.

The dominance deviation represents within locus interaction. It reflects the effect of putting genes together in pairs to make the genotypes. Dominance deviation may be obtained from the assumed genotypic values 'a' and 'd' by subtraction of breeding vale from genotypic value as shown in the Table below.

Dominance deviation

Population mean $(M) = a(p - q) + 2pqd$

Average effect of a gene $= \alpha = a + d(q - p)$

Therefore, $a = \alpha - d(q - p)$

Genotypes	A_1A_1	A_1A_2	A_2A_2
Genotype frequencies	p^2	$2pq$	q^2
Assigned value	a	d	−a
Genotypic value (G)	$2q(a - pd)$ $= 2q(\alpha - qd)$	$a(q - p) + d(1 - 2pq)$ $= (q - p)\alpha + 2pqd$	$-2p(a + qd)$ $= -2p(\alpha + pd)$
Breeding value (A)	$2q\alpha$	$(q - p)\alpha$	$-2p\alpha$
Dominance deviation $(D = G - A)$	$-2q^2d$	$2pqd$	$-2p^2d$

The assigned genotypic value to the genotype A_1A_1 is +a and the population mean $M = a(p - q) + 2pqd$. Therefore, the genotypic value of A_1A_1, expressed as a deviation from the population mean, is:

$$
\begin{aligned}
\text{Genotypic value of } A_1A_1 \ &= \ a - [a(p - q) + 2pqd] \\
&= \ a - [ap - aq + 2pqd] \\
&= \ a - ap + aq - 2pqd \\
&= \ a(1 - p + q) - 2pqd, \text{ by taking a as common} \\
&= \ a(q + q) - 2pqd \text{ since } 1 - p = q \\
&= \ a(2q) - 2pqd \\
&= \ 2q(a - dp) \text{ by taking 2q as common}
\end{aligned}
$$

This equation may be expressed in terms of the average of gene substitution, by substituting $a - d (q - p)$, as shown:

$$= 2q [\alpha - d (q - p) - dp]$$
$$= 2q [\alpha - dq + dp - dp]$$
$$= 2q [\alpha - dq], \text{ by striking out } +dp \text{ and } -dp$$
$$= 2q (\alpha - qd)$$

By subtracting the breeding value (A) from the genotypic value (G), the dominance deviation (D) may be obtained as shown:

$$D = G - A$$
$$= 2q (\alpha - qd) - 2q\alpha$$
$$= 2q\alpha - 2q^2d - 2q\alpha$$
$$= -2q\alpha, \text{ by striking out } 2q\alpha \text{ and } -2q\alpha$$

In a similar way, the dominance deviation of the genotypes A_1A_2 and A_2A_2 genotypes may be obtained as $2pqd$ and $-2p^2d$, respectively.

It may be observed that the dominance deviation of the three genotypes A_1A_1, A_1A_2 and A_2A_2 are the functions of d. If there is no dominance, the value becomes zero and all dominance deviations will be zero. Therefore, in the absence of dominance, the breeding value (A) and genotypic value (G) will be the same, i.e. $G = A$.

CLASS WORK

Based on the previous exercise, calculate the genotypic value (G), breeding value (A) and dominance deviation (D), when frequency of the pygmy gene (q) is 0.1.

$q = 0.1$, therefore, $p = 1.0 - 0.1 = 0.9$

Genotypes:	Pg Pg	Pg pg	pg pg
Frequency	0.81	0.18	0.01
G	0.44	−1.56	−7.56
A	0.48	−1.92	−4.32
D = G − A	−0.04	0.36	−3.24

Practical No. 9

9.1 ESTIMATION OF HERITABILITY BY HALF SIB METHOD

Heritability (h_B^2), in broad sense, is the ratio of genotypic value to the phenotypic variance, and it describes what proportion of the total phenotypic variance is due to the genotypic differences between the individuals in the population. This is given by:

$$h_B^2 = \frac{V_G}{V_P} = \frac{V_A + V_D + V_I}{V_A + V_D + V_I + V_E}$$

The broad sense heritability is not transmitted since the dominant and epistatic gene combinations are broken due to random segregation and recombination of genes in each generation.

Heritability in narrow sense (h_N^2) is defined as the ratio of additive genetic variance to the total phenotypic variance. It is given by:

$$h_N^2 = \frac{V_A}{V_P} = \frac{V_A}{V_A + V_D + V_I + V_E}$$

This fraction of heritability is transmitted in full to the next generation.

In general, the heritability estimates ranging from 10% to 20% are regarded as low heritability, 25% to 45% as moderate heritability and from 50% to 70% as high heritability. The traits related to fertility, fitness, health and survival have low heritabilities. Product quality traits such as fat and protein percentage tend to have the highest heritabilities.

METHODS OF ESTIMATION OF HERITABILITY

The following methods are commonly used to estimate the heritability in livestock breeding:

1. *Half-sib analysis*: This method is useful for uniparous animals with a longer generation interval like cattle. Each sire is mated to several dams and each dam produces one progeny. The data are recorded on the progeny, as half-sib groups.

2. *Full-sib analysis*: This method is useful for the livestock species that are highly prolific with a shorter generation interval like poultry and swine. In this method, each sire is mated to a group of dams and each dam produces a number of progeny and the data are recorded on

progeny as full sib groups. Data obtained from such mating are known as nested or hierarchical data.

3. *Regression of offspring on parent*: This method is useful for estimating the sire-son and sire-daughter regressions when a sire is mated to a series of dams and each dam has one progeny.

4. *Heritability estimation from selection experiments*: It is also known as realized heritability. It is based on the actual genetic gain, and it is not an expected estimate.

$$\text{Realized heritability} = \frac{\text{Response to selection (R)}}{\text{Selection differential (S)}}$$

A. Equal Number of Progeny per Sire:

Each sire is mated to a number of dams, and each produce single progeny and the data are recorded on the progeny as half-sib groups. The method described below is valid when the number of progeny per sire and number of dams per sire are equal.

Statistical Model:

$$Y_{ij} = \mu + S_i + e_{ij}, \text{ where,}$$
Y_{ij} = Observation on j^{th} progeny belonging to i^{th} sire
μ = Overall mean
S_i = Effect of ith sire
e_{ij} = Random error

The data are arranged in the form of half sib groups as:

		Sires		
		A	B	C
Progeny	1	Y_{11}	Y_{21}	Y_{31}
	2	Y_{21}	Y_{22}	Y_{23}
	3	Y_{31}	Y_{32}	Y_{33}
Total		$Y_{1.}$	$Y_{2.}$	$Y_{3.}$
N		3	3	3

$$Y.. = \text{Grand Total} = Y_{1.} + Y_{2.} + Y_{3.}$$
$$N = \text{Total number of observations} = 9$$
$$\text{Correction Factor (CF)} = \frac{(Y..)^2}{N}$$

Total Sum of Squares (TSS) crude $= \Sigma\Sigma\, (Y_{ij}{}^2)$

Total Sum of Squares (TSS) corrected $= (Y_{11})^2 + (Y_{21})^2 + \ldots + (Y_{33})^2 - CF$

Sum of squares between sires $= \sum \dfrac{(Y_i)^2}{n_i} - CF$

Sum of squares between progeny within sires (Error SS)

$$= \sum Y_{ij}^2 - \sum \frac{(Y_i)^2}{n}$$

The results are to be presented in the Analysis of Variance (ANOVA) Table as below.

ANOVA Table

Source of variation	d.f	Sum of Squares (SS)	Mean Squares (S)	Expected Mean Squares
Between sires	$(S-1)$	SS_S	$SS_S/(S-1)$	$\sigma^2_e + K\,\sigma^2_S$
Between progeny within sires	$(N-S)$	SS_e	$SS_e/(N-S)$	σ^2_e
Total	$(N-1)$	TSS		

S = Number of sires

N = Total number of progeny

σ^2_S = Sire component of variance

σ^2_e = Error component of variance

K = Average number of progeny per sire

Genetic variance $(\sigma_s 2) = \dfrac{MS_S - MS_e}{K}$

Intra-class correlation $(t) = (\sigma^2_S)/(\sigma^2_S + \sigma^2_e)$

Heritability $(h^2) = 4t$

The half sib correlation method estimates only 1/4th of the additive genetic variance and so, it must be multiplied by four to get total additive genetic variance.

CLASS WORK

1   In a Deoni cattle breeding farm, five sires were each mated to five dams and the daily milk yield (kg) one daughter from each dam were recorded as detailed below. Estimate the heritability of daily milk yield along with its standard error and offer your comments

	Sire A	Sire B	Sire C	Sire D	Sire E
Daughter 1	4.1	2.2	2.2	3.2	3.0
Daughter 2	4.0	3.2	3.0	4.0	5.0
Daughter 3	4.1	4.0	2.1	4.1	4.1
Daughter 4	3.2	3.0	3.1	2.2	2.1
Daughter 5	5.0	2.1	5.0	1.0	4.0
N	5	5	5	5	5
Sum	20.4	14.5	15.4	14.5	18.2
SS	84.86	44.49	52.86	48.89	71.22
Mean	4.08	2.9	3.08	2.9	3.64

S = Number of sires = 5

D = Number of dams = 5

K = Number of progeny per sire = 5

N = Total number of progeny = 25

Grand total (GT) = $4.1 + 4.0 + ... + 2.1 + 4.0 = 83.00$

Total Sum of Squares (crude/uncorrected) = $4.1^2 + 4.0^2 + ... + 4.0^2 = 302.32$

Correction Factor (CF) = $(GT)^2/N = (83.00)^2/25 = 275.56$

Total Sum of Squares (corrected) = TSS crude – Correction Factor

$$= 302.32 - 275.56 = 26.76$$

Sum of squares between sires

$$= [(20.4)^2/5 + (14.5)^2/5 + ... + (18.2)^2/5] - 275.56$$
$$= 1405.06/5 - 275.56$$
$$= 281.01 - 275.56 = 5.45$$

Sum of squares within sires or

Error sum of squares = TSS (corrected) − SS between sires
$$= 26.76 - 5.45 = 21.31 \text{ or}$$
$$= \text{TSS (crude)} - \text{SS between sires (crude)}$$
$$= 302.32 - 281.01 = 21.31$$

These results are presented in the following ANOVA Table:

ANOVA Table

Source of variation	d.f	Sum of Squares (SS)	Mean Sum of Squares (MS)	Expected Mean Squares (EMS)
Between sires	(S − 1) = 5 − 1 = 4	5.45	5.45/4= 1.36 (MS$_S$)	$\sigma^2_e + K \sigma^2_s$
Within sires (Error)	(N − S) = 25 − 5 = 20	21.31	21.31/20 = 1.07 (MS$_e$)	σ^2_e
Total	(N − 1) = 25 − 1 = 24	26.76		

Estimation of components of variance:

Genetic variance $(\sigma^2_S) = \dfrac{\text{MS}_S - \text{MS}_e}{K}$

Where, K = Average number of progeny per sire

$$= \frac{1.36 - 1.07}{5} = 0.058$$

Intra-class correlation (t) = $(\sigma^2_S)/(\sigma^2_S + \sigma^2_e)$
$$= 0.058/(0.058+1.07)$$
$$= 0.051$$

Heritability = 4t
$$= 4 \times 0.051 = 0.204$$

SE (h²) = 4 × √[2 (N − 1) (1 − t)²][1 + (K − 1)t]²/K² (N − S) (S − 1)

Where,

N = Total number of progeny = 25

S = Number of sires = 5

t = Intra-class correlation = 0.051

K = Number of progeny per sire = 5

After substituting the values in the above equation,

$$SE (h^2) = 4 \times \sqrt{[2 (25 - 1) (1 - 0.051)^2]}$$
$$[1 + (5 - 1)0.051]2/52 (25 - 5) (5 - 1)$$
$$= 4 \times \sqrt{0.0333}$$
$$= 4 \times 0.182$$
$$= 0.728$$

Therefore, the heritability of daily milk yield is 0.204 ± 0.728. The SE of the estimate is high which may be due to lower number of daughters per sires. The number of daughters per sire sample (5) in the present example is insufficient to establish the real genetic differences between the sires. The reliability of an estimate with larger SE is less.

2. In a Murrah buffalo herd, three sires were each mated to different number of dams, and each dam produced one calf. The data on birth weight of the calves are given below. Estimate the heritability of birth weight of the calves.

Calves	Sires		
	A	B	C
1	20	22	22
2	19	24	20
3	21	22	–
4	–	20	–
Total	60	88	42

Grand Total (GT) = 190; Total no. of observations = N = 9
Total Sum of Squares (crude/uncorrected) = $20^2 + 19^2 + \ldots + 20^2 = 4030$
Correction Factor (CF) = $(GT)^2/N = (190)^2/9 = 4011.11$
Total Sum of Squares (corrected) = TSS crude − Correction Factor
$$= 4030.00 - 4011.11 = 18.89$$
Sum of squares between sires = $[(60)^2/3 + (88)^2/4 + (42)^2/2] - 4011.11$
$$= 4018.00 - 4011.11 = 6.89$$
Sum of squares within sires or
Error sum of squares = TSS (corrected) − SS between sires
$$= 18.89 - 6.89 = 12.00 \text{ or}$$
$$= TSS \text{ (crude)} - SS \text{ between sires (crude)}$$
$$= 4030.00 - 4018.00 = 12.00$$

Theses results are presented in the following ANOVA Table:

ANOVA Table

	d.f	Sum of Squares (SS)	Mean Sum of Squares (MS)	Expected Mean Squares (EMS)
Between sires	$(S-1) = 3 - 1 = 2$	6.89	$6.89/2 = 3.45$	$\sigma^2_e + K\sigma^2_s$
Within sires (Error)	$(N-S) = 9 - 3 = 6$	12.00	$12.00/6 = 2.00$	σ^2_e
Total	$(N-1) = 9 - 1 = 8$	18.89		

Estimation of components of variance:

$$\text{Genetic variance } (\sigma^2 S) = \frac{MS_S - MS_e}{K} \text{ where,}$$

K = Average number of progeny per sire. When the number of progeny per sire is unequal, the K value may be computed as:

$$K = \frac{1}{(S-1)}\left(n - \frac{\sum n_i^2}{n}\right)$$

$$= \frac{1}{(3-1)}\left(9 - \frac{3^2 - 4^2 + 2^2}{9}\right)$$

$$= 2.89$$

$$\text{Genetic variance } (\sigma^2 S) = \frac{MS_S - MS_e}{K}$$

$$= \frac{3.45 - 2.00}{2.89}$$

$$\text{Intra-class correlation } (t) = (\sigma^2_s)/(\sigma^2_s + (\sigma^2_e)$$

$$= 0.43/(0.43 + 2.00)$$

$$= 0.18$$

$$\text{Heritability} = 4t$$

$$= 4 \times 0.18 = 0.72$$

3. In a population genetics study, the variances due to dominance deviation, epistatic effects and total genotypic effects for the weaning weight in a group of mice were 10, 5 and 60 kg², respectively. The environmental variance was 80 kg. Estimate the heritability of weaning weight.

$$\sigma^2_P = \sigma^2_G + \sigma^2_E$$
$$= 60 + 80 = 140$$

Similarly,

$$\sigma^2_G = \sigma^2_A + \sigma^2_D + \sigma^2_I$$
$$60 = \sigma^2_A + 10 + 5$$

Therefore,

$$\sigma^2_A = 60 - 10 - 5 = 45$$
$$h^2 \text{ (narrow sense)} = \sigma^2_A / \sigma^2_P = 45/140 = 0.32$$

The heritability of weaning weight is 0.32 or 32%. This indicates that 32% of the total phenotypic variation is due to genetic differences between the sires and the remaining 68% is attributed to non-genetic differences. Therefore, this trait can be considered for improvement through selection of the best sires for further propagation and genetic improvement.

HOME WORK

9.1.1 The number of services required for conception of nine Murrah buffaloes belonging to three sires are given below. Estimate the heritability along with its standard error.

	Sires		
	1	2	3
No. of services	2	6	3
per conception	3	2	7
of daughters	4	7	11

9.1.2 The first clip greasy fleece wool yield (kg) of a total 16 Deccani ewes, belonging to four different sires are given below. Calculate the heritability and offer your comments on the estimate obtained. (Ans: 0.84)

	Sires			
	P	Q	R	S
Wool Yield (kg)	2.8	2.6	1.9	2.8
	2.2	1.9	1.8	2.3
	1.7	1.8	2.0	2.6
	2.3	2.2	2.1	2.2

9.1.3   The data on egg weight (g) of 40 white Leghorn layers at 25 weeks of age, belonging to five sires, are given below. Estimate the heritability of egg weight and offer your comments on the estimate obtained. (Ans: 0.36)

	Sires				
	A	B	C	D	E
Egg weight of daughters (g)	55	57	54	45	54
	58	50	58	52	55
	57	48	53	49	59
	46	54	54	46	52
	53	56	56	50	60
	45	45	57	56	53
	–	55	59	50	48
	–	57	48	–	56
	–	54	53	–	–
	–	59	–	–	–

9.1.4   In a Murrah-buffalo-breeding farm, five sires were each mated with six dams. One cow from each mating was chosen randomly and the average butter fat percentage was recorded during first month of calving, which is detailed in the following Table. Calculate the heritability along with the Standard Error and offer your comments on the estimate obtained.

	Sire I	Sire II	Sire III	Sire IV	Sire V
	6.2	6.0	6.2	7.2	6.9
	6.9	6.6	6.8	6.6	6.9
Daughters'	7.6	6.7	5.9	6.7	7.9
butter fat%	7.5	6.1	6.8	6.1	6.8
	6.8	7.2	6.3	6.8	7.0
	7.4	6.9	6.9	7.9	7.5

9.1.5 There was a large herd of crossbred cattle. Five sires were each mated to eight dams and one progeny was chosen at random and their six months body weights (kg) were recorded. Estimate the heritability along with the standard error.

Sire no.	Progeny no.							
	1	2	3	4	5	6	7	8
1	68.7	69.1	79.3	67.5	70.0	79.3	70.4	71.4
2	61.8	68.0	59.2	68.3	63.1	69.1	69.4	73.2
3	61.8	68.7	76.3	74.7	67.8	73.7	73.1	66.3
4	60.0	65.7	66.9	60.6	71.8	69.3	66.9	64.8
5	71.7	65.8	67.4	61.1	67.8	78.8	65.0	69.0

9.1.6 The data recorded on clean fleece yield (kg) of a total of 16 Mandya ewes, belonging to four sires are given below. Estimate the heritability along with its standard error.

S_1	S_2	S_3	S_4
1.6	0.9	1.9	1.6
1.3	0.8	1.2	0.9
1.4	1.0	0.7	0.8
1.2	1.1	1.3	1.2

9.1.7 Calculate the heritability of days to attain peak yield (in months) of 12 Murrah buffaloes from the data on first three lactations given below.

S$_1$	S$_2$	S$_3$	S$_4$
4	3	2	3
4	2	4	2
3	3	3	3

9.1.8 Three boars were mated to five sows. The male progeny from each specific mating was chosen for recording backfat thickness in centimeters at 6 months of age. Calculate the heritability.

	Sire 1	Sire 2	Sire 3
	3.7	3.2	3.6
	3.6	3.3	3.5
Progeny	3.5	3.1	3.8
	3.8	3.7	3.6
	4.0	3.9	3.9

9.1.9 In a Sahiwal cattle herd, there were three sires, each mated to different number of dams, producing one calf each. Birth weights of calves were recorded in kilogram as given below. Calculate heritability of birth weight along with its standard error.

Sire 1	Sire 2	Sire 3
15	18	16
16	20	18
17	18	–
–	16	–

9.1.10 Average weaning weight (kg) of 100 lambs belonging to Hampshire cross from 15 sires was put to analysis of variance, sum of squares and degrees of freedom for different sources as given below. Calculate heritability by half sib method.

Source of variation	d.f.	SS	MSS
Between sires	14	429774.8	30698.20
Within sires	85	1304673.5	15349.10
Total			

9.1.11 The following data pertain to the age at sexual maturity of White leghorn progeny in an experiment. Estimate the heritability along with its standard error.

Sire no.	Progeny ASM (days)
1	129, 170, 141, 145, 159, 141, 151, 152, 139, 141, 151, 141, 124, 130, 136, 127
2	165, 123, 148, 149, 148, 156, 166, 145, 154, 152, 146, 140, 134, 145, 165, 145, 141
3	154, 143, 150, 163, 152, 167, 130, 152, 157, 144, 156, 136, 163, 164, 141, 153, 148, 140

9.2 ESTIMATION OF HERITABILITY BY FULL SIB METHOD

This method is commonly used in poultry, swine breeding and other litter-bearing animals like rabbits, which have a shorter generation interval. The data used for full sib analysis are hierarchical, in which every observation of the available data falls under a class, which itself, is a sub-class of a bigger classification, which in turn may be sub-classification of still larger classification. For example, in a breeding farm, 8 sires were each mated to a random sample of 5 dams and from each dam, 3 progeny are evaluated. Therefore, there are $8 \times 5 \times 3 = 120$ progeny to be studied under 40 dam classes, which are under 8 sire classes.

CLASS WORK

1. The data on individual body weights of bunnies (young rabbits) at 6 weeks age (g) were obtained from a rabbit-breeding farm. Five sires were each mated to three dams and each dam produced three progeny. The body weights of progeny were recorded and presented below. Estimate the heritability from sire, dam and sire + dam components of variance.

Sire no.	Dam no.	Progeny 1	Progeny 2	Progeny 3	Dam total	Sire total
1	1	553	500	609	1662	
	2	609	547	401	1557	4798
	3	641	498	440	1579	
2	4	637	635	587	1859	
	5	475	456	509	1440	5007
	6	625	511	572	1707	
3	7	496	532	386	1414	
	8	439	563	452	1454	4271
	9	500	507	396	1403	
4	10	465	421	497	1383	
	11	470	580	605	1655	4703
	12	488	498	679	1655	

	13	414	340	503	1257	
5	14	305	453	344	1102	4002
	15	465	513	665	1643	

Grand Total = 553 + 500 + ... + 513 + 665 = 22781

TSS (crude) = $553^2 + 500^2 + ... + 513^2 + 665^2$ = 11880279

S	= No. of sires = 5
D	= No. of dams = 15
N	= Total no. of progeny = 15 × 3 = 45
K_1 = No. of dams/sire	= 3
K_2 = No. of progeny/dam	= 3 (i.e., $K_1 = K_2$)
K_3 = No. of progeny/sire	= 3 dams × 3 progeny/dam = 9
Correction Factor (CF)	= (Grand Total)^2/N
	= $(22781)^2$/45
	= 11532754.69
TSS crude	= 11880279
TSS corrected	= TSS crude − CF
	= 11880279.00 − 11532754.69
	= 347524.31

Sum of Squares between sires (SS_S)

$$= \frac{(4798)^2 + (5007)^2 + ... + (4002)^2}{3} - CF$$

$$= 11607389.67 - 11532754.69$$

$$= 74634.98$$

Sum of Squares between sires (SS_D)

$$= \frac{(1662^2 + 1557^2 + ... + 1102^2 + 1643)^2}{3} - \text{Crude SS between sires}$$

= 11708747 − 11607389.67 = 101357.33

Sum of Squares between progeny
within dams within sires (Error SS)

= TSS corrected − (SS between sires + SS between dams)

= 347524.31 − (74634.98 + 101357.33) = 171532

Analysis of variance Table is computed for estimating the components of variance, as detailed below.

ANOVA Table

Source of variation	d.f	Sum of Squares (SS)	Mean Sum of Squares (MS)	Expected Mean Squares (EMS)
Between sires	$(S - 1) =$ $5 - 1 = 4$	74634.98	$74634.98/4 =$ 18658.75	$\sigma^2_W + K_2\sigma^2_D$ $+ K_3\sigma^2_S$
Between dams within sires	$(D - S) =$ $15 - 5 =$ 10	101357.33	$101357.33/10$ $= 10135.73$	$\sigma^2_W + K_1\sigma^2_D$
Between progeny within dams within sires (Error SS)	$(N - D)$ $= 45 - 15$ $= 30$	171532.00	$171532.00/30$ $= 5717.73$	σ^2_W
Total	$(N - 1) =$ $45 - 1 =$ 44			

Estimation of components of variance:

Error variance (σ^2_W) = MSW = 5717.73

$$\text{Dam variance } (\sigma^2_D) = \frac{MS_D - MS_W}{K_1} = \frac{10135.73 - 5717.73}{3}$$

$$= 1472.67$$

$$\text{Sire variance } (\sigma_S2) = \frac{MS_S - MS_D}{K_3} = \frac{18658.75 - 10135.73}{9}$$

$$= 947.00$$

Phenotypic variance $(\sigma^2_P) = \sigma^2_S + \sigma^2_D + \sigma^2_W$

$$= 947.00 + 1472.67 + 5717.73$$

$$= 8137.40$$

Heritability based on sire component $(h^2_S) = \dfrac{4\sigma^2_S}{\sigma^2_P} = \dfrac{4 \times 947.00}{8137.40} = 0.47$

Heritability based on dam component $(h_D^2) = \dfrac{4\sigma_D^2}{\sigma_P^2} = \dfrac{4 \times 1472.67}{8137.40}$
$= 0.72$

Heritability based on sire+dam component $(h_{S+D}^2) = \dfrac{2(\sigma_S^2 + \sigma_D^2)}{\sigma_P^2}$

$= \dfrac{2(947.00 + 1472.67)}{8137.40} = 0.595$

In general, heritability based on dam component (0.72) is highest due to maternal and sex-linked effects, based on sire component lowest while the sire + dam component heritability is intermediate.

HOME WORK

9.2.1   The data on egg weight (g) at 40 weeks of age in a strain of white Leghorns were obtained randomly. There were a total of 41 sires, each mated to 3 dams, producing 3 viable female progeny per dam. Estimate the heritability by all three components based on the following ANOVA Table.

ANOVA TABLE

Source of variation	d.f	SS	MSS
Between sires	40	954.00	23.85
Between dams within sires	82	1316.92	16.06
Between progeny within dams within sires	242	1979.56	8.16

9.2.2   The data on litter size at weaning of 27 large White Yorkshire sows born to 9 dams mated to 3 sires are given below. Estimate the heritability based on sire, dam and sire + dam components of variance.

Sires	Dams	Progeny litter size			Dam total	Sire total
1	1	4	5	6	15	
	2	5	8	5	18	
	3	4	6	8	18	51
2	4	5	6	9	20	
	5	9	8	7	24	
	6	4	4	8	16	60
3	7	7	6	9	22	
	8	8	9	8	25	
	9	7	5	6	18	65

9.2.3   The following data pertain to the age at sexual maturity in days
        of the progeny in a full sib experiment, in which each of the three
        sires were mated to 4 dams. Estimate the heritability.

Sires	Dams	Progeny ASM (days)				
1	1	129	170	141	145	–
	2	159	141	151	152	139
	3	141	151	141	–	–
	4	124	130	136	127	–
2	1	165	133	148	149	–
	2	148	156	166	145	154
	3	152	146	140	–	–
	4	134	145	165	145	141
3	1	154	143	150	163	–
	2	152	167	130	152	157
	3	144	156	136	163	164
	4	141	153	148	140	–

PRACTICAL NO. 10

10.1 ESTIMATION OF REPEATABILITY

Repeatability (r) is defined as the repetition of same trait several times in the lifetime of an individual. It can also be defined as the ratio of genotypic variance plus permanent environmental effect to the sum of genotypic variance, permanent environmental effects and temporary environmental effects. The permanent environmental effects are common to repeated measures and stay with the animal throughout its life but not passed onto the offspring. For example, loss of a leg due to accident, permanent udder damage, etc. The temporary environmental effects are specific for a particular measurement, and the effect is different in next measurement; for example, effect of season, year, etc. Repeatability can be estimated by the formula:

$$ r = \frac{V_G + V_{EP}}{V_G + V_{EP} + V_{ET}} $$

Repeatability ranges from zero to one. The larger the temporary environmental effects, the lower will be the repeatability.

Uses of repeatability

- Repeatability is an upper limit of the heritability of a trait. Therefore, in the absence of heritability, by seeing the repeatability, we can assess the heritability.

$$ r = \frac{V_G + V_{EP}}{V_G + V_{EP} + V_{ET}}, \text{ whereas } h^2 = \frac{V_A}{V_P} $$

- Repeatability can be used to determine increase in response with additional measures. Repeated measures help reduce the phenotypic variance, as the temporary environmental effects tend to cancel out.
- Repeatability can be used to estimate the future production of an animal on the basis of her past performance, using the formula for Most Probable Producing Ability (MPPA).

$$ \text{MPPA} = \frac{nr}{1 + (n-1)r} $$

Where, n is the number of records and r is the repeatability of the trait.

- For highly repeatable traits, the measurements are similar and so, additional measurements add little additional information. This results in small additional increase in response.
- For lowly repeatable traits, the measurements vary, and so, additional measurements add much additional information, as shown in the following table.

	n = 2	n = 5
r = 0.10	35%	89%
r = 0.50	16%	29%
r = 0.90	2.6%	4.3%

Estimates of repeatability

In general, the repeatability of some of the traits are:

Trait	r
Milk yield in dairy cattle	0.55
Weaning weight in calves	0.37
Greasy fleece weight in sheep	0.58
Wool fiber diameter in sheep	0.70

CLASS WORK

In a flock of Mandya sheep six animals were chosen at random and the staple length measurements (in cm) were recorded 10 times during their lifetime. Estimate the repeatability of staple length.

	Animal no.					
	A	B	C	D	E	F
Staple length (cm)	4.0	4.1	4.3	4.1	4.2	4.3
	3.9	4.0	4.4	4.6	4.1	4.2
	4.6	4.2	4.2	4.7	4.7	4.2
	4.5	4.0	4.6	4.0	4.2	4.0
	4.3	4.0	4.0	3.9	4.5	4.4
	4.0	3.8	3.7	3.9	4.6	4.8
	4.5	4.0	4.4	3.8	4.9	4.6
	4.2	3.7	4.1	4.3	4.3	4.5
	4.0	3.8	4.5	4.1	4.2	4.2
	3.7	3.7	4.7	4.2	5.0	4.3
Total	41.7	39.3	42.9	41.6	44.7	43.5

Total no. of animals (N)   = 6

Total no. of measurements   = 6 × 10 = 60

Grand total (GT)   = 4.0 + 3.9 + ... + 4.2 + 4.3

                                                            = 253.7

Total Sum of Squares (TSS) crude   = $4.0^2 + 3.9^2 + ... + 4.2^2 + 4.3^2$

                                                            = 1078.55

Correction Factor (CF)   = $(GT)^2 - CF$

                                                            = 1072.73

Total Sum of Squares (TSS) corrected = TSS crude − CF

                                                            = 1078.55 − 1072.73

                                                            = 5.82

SS between animals (SS_b) = $\dfrac{41.7^2 + 29.3^2 + ... + 44.7^2 + 43.5^2}{10}$ − CF

                                            = 1.74

SS within animals (SS_w) = TSS corrected − SS between animals

                                            = 5.82 − 1.74

                                            = 4.08

The results are presented in the ANOVA Table for further calculations.

Source of Variation	d.f	Sum of Squares	Mean Sum of Squares	Expected Mean Squares
Between animals	6 − 1 = 5	1.74	1.74 / 5 = 0.348 (MS_b)	$\sigma^2_w + K \sigma^2_b$
Within animals	60 − 6 = 54	4.08	4.08 / 54 = 0.076 (MS_w)	σ^2_w
Total	60 − 1 = 59			

From the above ANOVA Table, the components of variance are estimated as:

$\sigma^2_w = \dfrac{MS_b - MS_w}{n}$, where n is the number of measurements per animal

$\dfrac{0.348 - 0.076}{10} = 0.272$

$$\sigma^2_{\text{w}} = MS_{\text{w}}$$

$$\text{Repeatability (r)} = \frac{\sigma^2_b}{\sigma^2_b + \sigma^2_w} = \frac{0.272}{0.0272 + 0.076} = 0.782$$

$$\text{SE of repeatability} = \frac{2(1-r^2)\,[1+(K-1)r]^2}{\sqrt{(K\,(K-1)(n-1)}}$$

Where, K is the number of animals and n is the number of measurements

$$\text{per animal} = \frac{2(1-0.782)^2[1+(6-1)0.782]^2}{6(6-1)(10-1)} = 0.09$$

Therefore, the repeatability obtained is 0.782 ± 0.09.

HOME WORK

10.1.1 The data on body weights at 3 months age of 5 New Zealand White does (in kg) during the first 3 kindlings are given below. Estimate the repeatability along with its standard error.

Kindling	Doe no.				
↓	1	2	3	4	5
First	0.9	1.1	1.4	1.1	1.3
Second	1.1	1.1	1.3	1.1	1.2
Third	1.0	0.9	0.8	1.2	1.0

10.1.2 Estimate the repeatability of number of services per conception of Deoni cows based on the data given in first three matings of four different cows.

Lactation	Cow no.			
↓	1	2	3	4
1	3	4	4	3
2	4	4	3	3
3	3	3	4	3

10.1.3 Estimate the repeatability of lactation milk yield (in 10 kg units) based on the data given on four Ongole cows in first three lactations.

Lactation	Cow no.			
↓	1	2	3	4
1	74	81	81	78
2	75	80	82	79
3	78	79	82	80

10.1.4 In a pig farm, five sows furrowed three times each and produced the following litter sizes at birth. Calculate the repeatability.

Sow	Litter size		
no. ↓	1	2	3
1	3	4	5
2	6	9	6
3	5	4	6
4	5	8	6
5	6	9	8

10.1.5 The data on litter size at birth of 25 Californian White does in five kindlings are given below. Estimate the repeatability.

Kindling	Does				
no. ↓	1	2	3	4	5
1	6	5	4	4	3
2	7	6	7	9	6
3	7	6	6	4	5
4	7	6	7	8	6
5	9	8	7	9	4

10.1.6 Estimate the repeatability of lactation milk yield based on the data given on four Ongole cows in four lactations (Milk yield is expressed in 10 kg units).

Lactation	Animal no.			
no. ↓	1	2	3	4
1	78	82	79	81
2	75	81	78	80
3	74	82	80	79

10.1.7 The litter size at the time of birth in first two furrowings of ten crossbred large White Yorkshire sows is given below. Estimate the repeatability along with its standard error.

Sow no. →	1	2	3	4	5	6	7	8	9	10
1st furrowing	11	9	13	10	9	8	10	11	10	13
2nd furrowing	10	12	12	10	8	6	12	9	12	12

10.1.8 The data on lactation milk yield (kg) for the same buffaloes mated to the same sires in four different lactations are given below. Estimate the repeatability.

Animal no.			
1	2	3	4
1501	1210	1400	1228
1386	1610	1360	1282
1430	1580	1290	1276
1422	1545	1385	1174
1370	–	–	–

PRACTICAL NO. 11

11.1 ESTIMATION OF GENETIC AND PHENOTYPIC CORRELATIONS

The correlation arising from genetic cause is called as genetic correlation while the correlation arising from common environmental cause is called environmental correlation. The observed correlation arising from the combined effects of genotypes and environment is known as phenotypic correlation. Genetic correlation is the association between two traits X and Y, which is due to additive gene effect. It arises mainly due to pleiotropy. However, linkage and heterozygosity may also cause genetic correlation but it is not stable.

If the genetic correlation is positive between two traits, selection for one trait will automatically brings about a change in the trait not selected for. For example, selection for feed efficiency in chickens will increase the average daily gain. Two or more traits may be genetically correlated negatively. In such case, selection for the improvement of one trait will result in decline in other trait. For example, selection for increased milk yield in dairy cattle will results in decreased butter fat percentage.

Two traits in an individual may be correlated because of the common environment. The environment correlation may be positive or negative.

CLASS WORK

1. The data on birth weight (X, in kg) and body length (Y, in cm) of nine calves belonging to 3 sires are given below. Estimate the genetic and phenotypic correlations.

Sire 1		Sire 2		Sire 3	
Birth weight (X)	Body length (Y)	Birth weight (X)	Body length (Y)	Birth weight (X)	Body length (Y)
18	50	15	30	16	40
20	60	16	40	18	50
18	50	17	50	–	–
16	40	–	–	–	–
72	200	48	120	34	90

(i) Estimation of components of variance for birth weight (X):

No. of observations (N) $= 4 + 3 + 2 = 9$

Grand total (GT) $= 72 + 48 + 34 = 154$

Total Sum of squares (uncorrected) $= 18^2 + 20^2 + ...+ 16^2 + 18^2$

$= 2654$

Correction Factor (CF) $= (GT)^2/N = (154)^2/9 = 2635.11$

Total Sum of squares (corrected) $=$ TSS uncorrected $-$ CF

$= 2654.00 - 2635.11$

$= 18.89$

Sum of Squares between sires (SS$_s$) $= \dfrac{72^2}{4} + \dfrac{48^2}{3} + \dfrac{34^2}{2} - CF$

$= 2642.00 - 2635.11$

$= 6.89$

Sum of Squares within sires (SS$_w$) $=$ TSS corrected $-$ SS$_s$

$= 18.89 - 6.89$

$= 12.00$

The components of variance of birth weight are calculated as:

Source of variation	d.f	SS	' MSS	EMS
Between sires	$(S - 1) = 3 - 1$ $= 2$	6.89	$6.89/2 = 3.45$ (MS$_s$)	$\sigma^2_w + K\,\sigma^2_s$
Within sires	$(N - S) = 9 - 3$ $= 6$	12.00	$12.00/6 = 2.00$ (MS$_w$)	σ^2_w
Total	$(N - 1) = 9 - 1$ $= 8$	18.89		

$$\sigma^2_S = \frac{MS_S - MS_W}{K},$$ where K is the average number of progeny per sire

Since the number of progeny per sire is unequal, the K value is computed as follows.

$$K = \frac{1}{(S-1)}\left(n. - \frac{\sum n_i^2}{n.}\right), \text{ where}$$

$S =$ Number of sires

n_i = Number of progeny per i^{th} sire

n. = Total number of progeny

$$K = \frac{1}{(3-1)}\left(9 - \frac{4^2 + 3^2 + 2^2}{9}\right)$$

$$\sigma_s^2 = \frac{3.45 - 2.00}{2.89} = 0.50$$

$$\sigma_w^2 = MS_w = 2.00$$

$$\sigma_p^2 = \sigma_s^2 + \sigma_w^2 = 0.50 + 2.00 = 2.50$$

(ii) Estimation of components of variance for body length (Y):

No. of observations (N)   = 4 + 3 + 2 = 9

Grand Total (GT)   = 200 + 120 + 90 = 410

Total Sum of squares (uncorrected)   = $50^2 + 60^2 + ...+ 40^2 + 50^2$

= 19300

Correction Factor (CF)   = $(GT)^2/N = (410)^2/9$

= 18677.78

Total Sum of squares (corrected)   = TSS uncorrected − CF

= 19300.00 − 18677.78

= 622.22

Sum of Squares between sires (SS_s) = $\dfrac{(200)^2}{4} + \dfrac{(120)^2}{3} + \dfrac{(90)^2}{2}$ − CF

= 18850.00 − 18677.78

= 172.22

Sum of Squares within sires (SS_w) = TSS corrected − SS_s

= 622.22 − 172.22

= 450.00

The components of variance of body length (Y) are calculated as:

Source of variation	d.f	SS	MSS	EMS
Between sires	(S − 1) = 3 − 1 = 2	172.22	172.22/2 = 86.11 (MS_s)	$\sigma_w^2 + K\,\sigma_s^2$
Within sires	(N − S) = 9 − 3 = 6	450.00	450.00/6 = 75.00 (MS_w)	σ_w^2
Total	(N − 1) = 9 − 1 = 8	622.22		

$$\sigma_S^2 = \frac{MS_S - MS_W}{K}, \text{ where K is the average number of progeny per}$$
sire

$$= \frac{86.11 - 75.00}{2.89}$$

$$\sigma_W^2 = MS_W = 75.00$$

$$\sigma_P^2 = \sigma_S^2 + \sigma_W^2 = 3.84 + 75.00 = 73.84$$

(iii) Estimation of the components of covariance between body weight and body length:

GT (body weight, X)   =   154.00

GT (body length, Y)   =   410.00

Total no. of observations (N)   =   9

$$\text{Correction Factor (CF)} = \frac{GT(X) \times GT(Y)}{N}$$

$$= \frac{154.00 \times 410.00}{9} = 7015.56$$

Total Sum of Cross Products (TSCP)

$$= (18 \times 50) + (20 \times 60) + \ldots + (18 \times 50)$$

$$= 7120.00$$

TSCP corrected = TSCP uncorrected − CF

$$= 7120.00 - 7015.56$$

$$= 104.44$$

Sum of Cross Products between sires (SCPs)

$$= \frac{(72 \times 200)}{4} + \frac{(48 \times 120)}{3} + \frac{34 \times 90}{2} - CF$$

$$= 7050.00 - 7015.56$$

$$= 34.44$$

Sum of Cross Products within sires = SCP − SCP_S

$$(SCP_W) = 104.44 - 3.44$$

$$= 70.00$$

The components of covariance of body weight and length are calculated as:

Source of variation	d.f	SCP	MSCP	EMCP
Between sires	$(S-1) = 3-1 = 2$	34.44	$34.44/2 = 17.22$ $(MSCP_S)$	$Cov_{(W)} + K$ $Cov_{(S)}$
Within sires	$(N-S) = 9-3 = 6$	70.00	$70.00/6 = 11.67$ $(MSCP_W)$	$Cov_{(W)}$
Total	$(N-1) = 9-1 = 8$	104.44		

$$Cov_S = \frac{MSCP_S - MSCP_W}{K}$$

$$\frac{17.22 - 11.67}{2.89} = 1.92$$

$$Cov_W = MSCP_W = 11.67$$

$$Cov_P = Cov_S + Cov_W = 1.92 + 11.67 = 13.59$$

(iv) Estimation of the genetic (r_g) and phenotypic correlations (r_p):

$$r_g = \frac{COV_S}{\text{Square root of } [(Var_S \text{ of body weight} \times Var_S \text{ of body length})]}$$

$$= \frac{1.92}{\text{Square root of } (0.50 \times 3.84)} = 1.38$$

$$r_p = \frac{COV_P}{\text{Square root of } (\sigma_P^2 \text{ of body weight} \times \sigma_P^2 \text{ of body length})}$$

$$= \frac{13.59}{\text{Square root of } (2.50 \times 73.84)} = 0.968$$

HOME WORK

11.1   The data on body weight at calving (X, in 100 kg units) and first lactation milk yield (Y, in 1000 kg units) of 18 Murrah buffaloes, belonging to three sires are given below. Estimate the genetic and phenotypic correlations.

Sires		Sire 1		Sire 2		Sire 3	
X		Y	X	Y	X	Y	
Progeny	1	3	2	5	3	4	3
	2	3	1	5	3	4	2
	3	4	3	3	1	2	1
	4	6	4	2	1	3	2
	5	6	5	3	2	3	1
	6	4	3	3	1	4	2
Sum		26	18	21	11	20	11
SS		122	64	81	25	70	23

11.2   Estimate the genetic and phenotypic correlations from the following ANOVA Table (K = 9.57).

Source of variation	d.f	MSS_X	$MSCP_{XY}$	MSS_Y
Between sires	69	638668.79	8700.86	2819.40
Within sires	657	326401.73	2810.52	2341.76
Total	726			

11.3   Calculate the genetic correlation between the age at conception (in 10 months units, X) and lactation milk yield (in 1000 kg units, Y), based on the data given below.

Progeny	Sire 1		Sire 2		Sire 3		Sire 4	
	X	Y	X	Y	X	Y	X	Y
1	3	3	4	3	3	3	3	3
2	4	4	3	3	4	2	3	3
3	3	4	2	2	4	4	2	2

11.4   The following data shows first lactation milk yield in 1000 kg units (Y) of the daughters of three sires with their corresponding body weights in 100 kg units (X) at first calving. Calculate the genetic and phenotypic correlations.

Sire 1		Sire 2		Sire 3	
Body weight (X)	LMY (Y)	Body weight (X)	LMY (Y)	Body weight (X)	LMY (Y)
4	3	5	3	3	2
4	2	5	3	3	1
2	1	3	1	4	3
3	2	2	1	6	4
3	1	3	2	6	5
4	2	3	1	4	3
–	–	3	2	4	2
–	–	–	–	3	1

11.5 The results of the analysis of variance and covariance of body weights of commercial broiler chickens at 4 and 6 weeks age and 4×6 weeks age are given below. Estimate the genetic, phenotypic and environmental correlations.

Source of variation	4-week body weight		6-weeks body weight		4 week × 6 week weight	
	d.f	MSS	d.f	MSS	d.f	MSCP
Between sires	27	8995.18	27	2050851.00	27	11269.59
Within sires	1551	1605.04	1497	4922.23	1497	1035.46
K1		56.1		54.2		54.2

Index

www.ingramcontent.com/pod-product-compliance
Lightning Source LLC
Chambersburg PA
CBHW061150220326
41599CB00025B/4435